VEGAN 1 Day

Stories of Living the Good Life

Foreword by Gene Baur, Co-Founder of Farm Sanctuary

VEGAN 1 Day

Stories of Living the Good Life

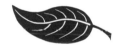

John Merryfield
Carol Merryfield

Contents

Foreword

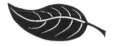

In affluent countries like the United States, we grow up eating meat, dairy and eggs, and unwittingly support abusive industries. Those industries, in fact, receive government subsidies that result in lower prices and more widespread consumption. We are bombarded by advertising that encourages us to consume animal products, and we ignore the myriad negative impacts of animal agriculture.

But, thankfully, that is beginning to change. With consumers learning more about the food they eat, the cruelty of factory farming and its destructive ecological impacts, and the benefits of eating plants instead of animals, a burgeoning vegan movement is taking root.

I am moved by the gentle wisdom that my friends John and Carol share in *Vegan 1 Day*, which inspires us to live according to our better angels. They reflect on their own aspirations and experiences, as well as the challenges we all face, struggling to make sense of this world. We are asked to

examine the ways our beliefs and actions shape our lives –
and our world – and we are encouraged to be mindful as we
strive to do better. It all begins with just one step, just one
day, and builds from there.

Being vegan is an aspiration to live as kindly as possible,
to stand against the exploitation and slaughter of other
animals and the squandering of our earth's precious
resources. It reflects a desire to live consciously and in
alignment with our own compassionate values, and to
breathe hope into a world marred by widespread cruelty and
destruction.

Killing animals is not only bad for them – it's also bad for
us. Can you imagine what it would be like to work in a
slaughterhouse? Doing so requires a person to turn off
their empathy. It also leads us to rationalize cruelty and
killing by denigrating our victims, as stupid or unworthy of
kindness, which ultimately degrades our own humanity
even further.

Shifting to a plant-based food system would alleviate
the unnecessary suffering of billions of animals and so much
more. Medical experts estimate that we could save 70%
on health care costs if our nation adopted a whole foods
plant-based diet. And, we could significantly lighten our
ecological footprint. The United Nations reports that
animal agriculture is one of the top contributors to our
planet's most serious environmental problems, including
climate change.

As individuals and as a species, we can learn from our
mistakes and make changes, or we can continue repeating
them. The harmful consequences of our animal based food
system are clear, as are the benefits of shifting to eating

plants instead. Every day, we make choices about what we eat that have profound impacts, which deserve our careful consideration. But where do we begin? Right here, right now, beginning with just one day.

Think about it. If we can live well without causing unnecessary harm, why wouldn't we?

Gene Baur

July 2016

Gene Baur is the president and co-founder of Farm Sanctuary and has been hailed as "the conscience of the food movement" by *Time* magazine. He is a longtime vegan, marathon runner, and Ironman triathlete, and national bestselling author of the book, *Farm Sanctuary: Changing Hearts and Minds About Animals and Food*, and co-author of the book, *Living the Farm Sanctuary Life: The Ultimate Guide to Eating Mindfully, Living Longer, and Feeling Better Every Day*.

Introduction

The compilation of stories in this book is a simple expression of this beautiful life we live. Ultimately, our hope is that you use this book as a guide to living a healthier, more authentic life that aligns with your core values; a life true to your own vision of good, your own idea of success, your own hope for a better world.

We are capable of so much more than we allow. Our journey is neither ordinary, nor extraordinary, and your path will not look exactly like ours. Our sincere hope is to inspire you along your own path, to find and experience the richness of a vegan way of life and to live in the beauty of one day at a time.

John and Carol

Carol's Story

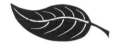

"Animals are my friends... and I don't eat my friends."

~ George Bernard Shaw

I was born into an Italian family that owned a restaurant in New York. It was a joint with a jukebox, counter service and some tables. It was right down the street from my junior high school, and I was able to go there for lunch. There was always a box and slips of paper to vote for your favorite Rheingold Girl. Rheingold was a popular beer back then and I always wrote a zillion slips for the one I thought should win.

Our restaurant served all kinds of burgers with fries, grilled cheese, tuna melts and BLT's. These are the typical foods I grew up on, along with lots of sweets and soda. In the 60's my father took on a partner who owned a cattle ranch in the mid-west. They changed the name of the restaurant to The Ranch, and it was all about steak and more steak.

Along with the restaurant food, there were always fresh meatballs every Sunday morning after Mass at my grandparent's house. There were manicotti, rigatoni, lasagna, baked ziti, sausage and peppers, and my favorite, cheese stuffed ravioli. There was every kind of antipasto and always salad with oil and vinegar.

I never thought about where my food came from, and had many emotional attachments to what I ate and when I ate it. There was always an agenda of which foods we ate at every occasion. At Christmas we always had ham, plus the pasta dishes. There was also a variety of Italian desserts, such as panettone, pizzelle, and other traditional Italian cookies. But my favorite was the struffoli, a traditional Christmas dessert made from small puffs of dough that are fried and dipped in honey and then sprinkled with colored candy. We always had at least two, and they were shaped like Christmas trees.

For the Fourth of July we always had a big cookout with hamburgers, hot dogs, chicken and pasta. At Easter it was ham again, and the pasta dishes, Easter bread and other desserts. At Thanksgiving it was the traditional turkey and fixings. It was comforting to know what to expect on these occasions. It was truly the meaning of comfort food, with all my family gathered together.

I moved away from New York to a mountain resort town in California when I was twenty-three. I had never eaten or even seen an avocado, and it seemed like avocados were everywhere in California!

When I was growing up we always had dogs and I had always considered myself an animal lover. At night my prayers consisted not only of prayers for my family and friends, but also my pets, and my friend's pets too. Our dog Butch was always at the top of the list even before family members, followed by other dogs, birds and turtles.

Husky, Bambi, Bruno, Daisy, Anoki, Kali, Dum and Dee, Homer and Jethro, and Jesse and Jeffrey. Then the prayer continued: If there are any lost animals, please let them be found. If they had good homes, let them be returned there safely without injury. If they had bad homes let them be returned somewhere else where they will be loved, happy and cherished for the rest of their lives, amen. I said this prayer every night, just that way.

After moving to California, I got a job at a European restaurant. They served every kind of meat you can imagine in rich sauces. Beef, lamb, duck, chicken and seafood. I worked there for many years eating these foods, never thinking anything about where my food came from. I called myself an animal lover, as my prayers confirmed, yet my entire life up to that point, I had been eating animals.

It's interesting for me to see young children now who have been brought up eating animals going to their first petting zoo or a farm. Some of them suddenly realize, oh, that's a chicken! That's what mommy cooked last night. There's a lamb! That's what we eat on Sunday? Many of us have been raised with this disconnect and easily pass it on to our children, just like I was. Some children are truly shocked and saddened by this, and although I was an adult when I made this connection, I too was shocked and saddened.

I met John in 1985, and in becoming friends he told me that he was a vegetarian. It was truly the first time I ever thought about what I was eating, and where my food came from. I started doing some research. I saw heartbreaking videos of factory farming and the utter disregard for the lives and feelings of these helpless animals. This is when I made the connection and in 1986, I became a vegetarian. It wasn't long after that we stopped eating eggs after realizing the cruelty in the egg industry. Egg-laying hens live lives of extreme confinement before being sent to slaughter.

If everyone on the planet went vegan for just 1 DAY, we would save -

- 68,493 egg-laying hens killed per day globally
- 68,493 baby male chicks killed per day globally (male chicks are an unwanted by-product of the egg industry)

(*Source: United Poultry Campaign*)

In 1999 when I started finding out the devastating and brutal practices of the dairy industry, I suggested to John that we should eliminate all dairy from our diet, and become vegans. He was all for the idea, but at that time, we weren't consistent in staying vegan. It seemed too easy to slip back into eating cheese once in a while and using butter. I didn't know how I was going to make the foods we liked without cheese, or bake without using butter. It wasn't until 2007 when we heard Erik Marcus, author of the book, *Meat Market: Animals, Ethics, and Money* that we were able to finally stick to being vegan.

Erik used charts and diagrams when speaking about the horrors of the dairy industry, and our motivation became very clear. Knowing that female cows were artificially inseminated over and over and over again, until they were depleted and that their babies were taken away at birth just completely broke my heart. This was devastating information and for me, it was a turning point.

The world is making more and more vegan products every day, and it's not so hard to live a vegan lifestyle anymore. Today we eat sweet potato stuffed ravioli, baked ziti, meatball wedges, donuts and cookies of all kinds. Every delicious food that we used to eat has been veganized! We recently had a vegan cannoli at Candle 79 in New York City. What more could a good Italian girl ask for? When John and I started the Vegan 1 Day Project we had no idea of the impact it might have. It has been a privilege to share the Vegan 1 Day message of compassion for animals and environmental sustainability with the community, while supporting John's one-day paddle around Lake Tahoe each year. Our potluck on the beach after the paddle has grown bigger each summer. This past year The Vegan 1 Day Project sponsored a showing of the amazing film *Cowspiracy* at our local theater. Speaking with people after the show, and by the phone calls we received the next day, we knew it made a huge impact.

Knowing that three times a day I can choose compassion in the foods I eat, and that no animal has been harmed for my meal, has made my life better in so many ways. I don't know anyone who has ever said that they support animal cruelty. Ask children what they want to be when they grow up, and many will say a veterinarian. All people naturally love animals, and want to help them. The more we raise the curtain on these incredibly cruel practices, the more people will change what they are eating.

Choosing kindness over cruelty makes the world a better place for all of us. The little girl that prayed every night for so many animals has now truly become an animal lover.

The life that John and I live is rooted in love: love

for each other; love for animals; love for the environment. It's a good life. The Vegan 1 Day Project is about helping people look at their own values of love and kindness, inspiring people to infuse their own values of love and kindness into their food choices one meal at a time. I hope the following stories that John wrote about our life together will inspire you to live the good life one day at a time.

The Green Flash

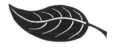

*"We desire to liberate and disassociate ourselves, as much
as possible, from the cruder forms of exploitation:
the plunder of the planet; the slavery of man and beast;
the slaughter of men in war, and of animuls for food"*
~ Scott and Helen Nearing *(Homesteading pioneers)*

Traveling across the sea like church bells, waves gather the
pieces of our fallen world to make beautiful things – sea
glass, driftwood, rounded stones, pieces of tile. We search
for some of these every morning on our walk along the beach
after sunrise.

It's been fourteen days in a row that we've sat in the
same spot on a small windswept mound of sand to watch
for the green flash. From the Sea of Cortez, just before the
sun gives birth to itself, there is the green flash and then it
is gone. The colored light travels faster than the sound of
a church bell traversing a calm ocean.

I am no longer in charge of positioning the blanket on
the beach in the morning. My haphazard placement lacks
my wife Carol's creative touch. Move it two or three inches
to the side, rotate it a bit, smooth the edges, bingo, it's
transformed into a home away from home. I hold our

two cups of tea as she designs and builds the morning nest with the beach towel for the sunrise.

Carol was the first to see the green flash and explained to me how to focus, or un-focus, my gaze on the horizon just where the sun comes up in order to recognize the quick, subtle flash of green light. The first time I saw it, it was lime green. Now sometimes, light blue. Before disappearing in a flash, the small burst of hazy color reminds me of a miniature Mark Rothko painting.

Whether or not I see the green flash isn't as important as sitting on the soft sand next to Carol in front of the Sea experiencing the gift of life.

This morning, sitting silently before the sunrise, we set our eyes to the horizon for the green flash. A solitary bee moves very slowly before us, struggling, and tumbling over in the sand. I reach over and offer my hand for the bee to climb onto. Just as I do, the bee gathers herself and flies away as if full of life and ready for the day. In the moment it takes to reach over with my hand, paying attention to the bee, the sun rises and we miss the green flash. Then we realize without any words spoken that helping the morning bee take flight is our green flash for the day.

The miracles of life surround us every day. There is joy, freedom and wonderment in living in the moment, and in every moment. But at times, we can get lost in the shuffle of life. We can become so focused on earning a living and meeting our obligations that we become cogs in a machine, leaving us uninspired and powerless to effect change in our lives, much less in the world that has gifted us life. Then, when on vacation, we'll sit by the proverbial pool in the sunshine, doing as little as possible while licking our wounds from the rough and tumble world. Just like the green flash, our lives are brief. The wondrous moment of our existence is here and then it is gone.

Carol and I live and work in Lake Tahoe six months a year, where we have grown children, and now grandchildren. The other six months out of the year, we live in Los Barriles, Baja, Mexico. In the USA, I work as a painting contractor, and Carol runs her business, The House Therapist. We earn a modest living, doing what we love. We don't live to work; we work to live. Our work is a means to an end.

Our goal every year in the USA is to spend as much time with family as possible and to make enough money to get back down to Baja for the season. We realize that this is not the most conventional of approaches to getting ahead and retiring with a comfortable nest egg.

Life is too short to short ourselves of the fullness it has to offer. We're more attracted to living a beautiful life, needing less, and doing something good in the world.

Living in Mexico half the year is a choice. We're choosing to live the dream of loving people and animals and the ocean and earth over the love of money and things. For us, it is a healthy alternative to getting ahead, making money, looking good, being busy, and braving the snow and cold of winter.

But it is more than that. It's a turning toward ourselves and toward all of life around us. It's a discovery of who we are and what is real to us again and again, season after season. We want to free ourselves of causing others harm due to our always wanting more. We want to be true to ourselves. We want to leave this world with more kindness and less cruelty, to give rather than take.

We are not wealthy people monetarily. Our wealth comes from the quality of life we have chosen to live. But nor are we living the lives of monastics under a palm tree off of the grid. We've found a happy medium balancing Carol's love for a creative home and my vision of simplicity.

Our travel every year down the Baja is a journey into the heart of Mexico where less is more and shedding the layers of stress and obligations is a process that starts in our own minds. Spending the winters in Baja is our form of rejuvenating our souls.

To live vegan is also one of the ways we honor the depth of our souls and the precious gift we have been given to live on this planet.

We've made the drive down the Baja highway more than twenty times. The van is always packed full of surfboards, books, quinoa, organic soy milk, and a few garage sale finds from the states, like chairs and dressers. Ex-pats in Mexico are called gringos, but many of us refer to each other as 'bringos' because we bring all of our stuff from the USA with us to Mexico.

Every season on the drive into Mexico, we notice the inventory we're bringing with us from the states. It's not so much the tangible items that get our attention; you can't miss all of the items loaded on top of the van. It's the intangibles—the subtle forms of stress, anxiety, competition, or other ways we're being untrue to ourselves—that come to mind.

Knowing what our truth is and living that truth has required a more nuanced awareness of ourselves. The drive into Mexico has, at times, provided interesting information about what we bring with us into our world.

We used to bring down several flats of Fuji apples, which we love and are hard to get in Baja. But this Fuji apple smuggling operation required me to stash the fruit-loot into the bottom of my wetsuit bag and avoid telling the truth at the agricultural inspection station in Guerrero Negro. Lying to a courteous, smiling Mexican agricultural inspector in the middle of the Baja desert made no sense at all and it felt silly. Besides, there is an abundance of existing fresh, organic, local fruit (much of it growing on trees in our neighborhood, including papaya, lime, mango, orange, lemon, and avocado).

So, giving up on Fuji apples hasn't been so difficult, but giving up on bending the rules to avoid consequences has proven more challenging.

My path of truth hit a tope (an omnipresent Baja speed bump) on this one particular drive down the Baja peninsula.

On the relatively easy last leg of the drive down the Baja, we arrived at Ciudad Constitucion just before noon. There was plenty of time to get home to Los Barriles before dark so I suggested that we stop at a roadside cart for a Mexican fruit cup, and at a cafe for a coffee drink. After finishing our delicious fruit cups of mango, watermelon, papaya, orange, jicama, coconut with salt, Chile powder and lime juice (no Fuji apples), we looked for a coffee shop.

On the other side of the street we noticed an American-style coffee shop with a convenient parking spot right in front. Perfect! Who doesn't love a parking spot right in front? Nice parking spots make us smile. It's one of the little things in life, but after 1,000 miles of the Baja highway a parking spot in the front of the coffee shop is a beautiful thing!

I ordered two single shot soy lattes to go; a nice treat for the easy cruise on home to Barriles. As I was walking out of the cafe, a Policia Municipal truck with two policemen pulled up alongside our van. The sight of la policia didn't give me concern, "Buenas... tardes." Hesitating, I looked at my watch to make sure it was actually afternoon and not before noon, which would have required a "Buenas Dias." They returned the "buenas tardes" greeting and then asked why I had parked in the handicap parking spot. Handicap parking spot?

Before answering, I scanned the area searching for some indication that it was a handicap parking spot. I squinted my eyes and craned my neck looking down to see the chipped away, barely visible, handicap parking blue color. It was the kind of blue paint that one might see on the side of a Mexican panga boat with fourteen applications of different colored paint layered on top.

I made a split second decision. It would have been senseless to engage in a conversation with la policia about the lack of adequate blue paint to sufficiently show tired road weary gringos, such as us, that it was indeed a handicap parking spot. Such a conversation would result in a "Mordida" (Mexican pay-off, bribe) and fewer Pesos in my wallet. Instead, I un-heroically thought of my wife and say, "Ah si, mi esposa, ella tiene un mal pierna" (Oh yeah, my wife, she has a bad leg) pointing to my own thigh.

Oh God, what the hell was I doing, I thought to myself. Even while speaking Spanish in that moment, I reminded myself of Rodney Dangerfield in Caddyshack, "Oh my arm, my arm, I think it's broken."

La policia responded, "Pues si, pero esta discapacidado"? (Yes, but is she handicapped?) I said, "No, she's not handicapped, but she can't walk very well," which is nowhere near the truth. And by the way, I thought to myself, where is my wife?

La policia maintained, "Puro estacionamiento discapacidad" (Only handicap parking). Still, I insisted that my wife was very injured and could barely walk.

Maybe it was my Spanish and ease of conversing, or a sense of leniency, but incredibly, the two policemen started nodding very slowly in acknowledgement and began pulling away ever so slowly. Had I avoided the mordida?

Just then, I noticed Carol up the street, with a healthy *giddy up - I've got a soy latte and we're almost home* stride to her step.

The conversation with la policia happened so fast, and I lied so easily. Carol was walking so briskly toward me with la policia still within eyeshot. What should I do?

"Carol," I yelled. "Hobble!"

As if right on cue I wanted her to act wounded and feeble. My expectations were ludicrous.

"What?" she asked, oblivious of my encounter with la policia and now walking straight for the van. Unbeknownst to me, when I was speaking to la policia, she was out of sight, crouched down, petting one of the town's stray dogs laying on the sidewalk.

"Hobble," I yelled again with more anxiety in my voice.

"What?" she replied again. She began acting more confused, even a little perturbed, with some of her New York Italian heritage becoming visible.

That's when it hit me, like a giant Fuji apple falling from the sky and landing on my head. Carol had no idea about this little charade I had been playing with la policia. Here she was now walking toward me with an irritated look on her face, and la policia still within sight. It goes without saying that lying is not the worst thing I've ever done in my life, but more to the point, lying is not who I am. Lying is not being true to myself.

This is me feeling the need to hustle my way through life, or that the rules don't apply to me, or whatever the root of getting away with something like this is.

Why do I bring the rat race with me to Mexico? I had, after all, parked in a handicap parking spot. I was in the wrong. There is a monetary fine for parking in Handicap parking spots. I should have paid whatever the mordida would have been. Wait. Let me modify that statement... I should have paid a fair, agreed upon, *negotiated* mordida!

Perhaps this entire charade I was playing with la policia might seem humorous, which it is, or maybe even too inconsequential to ruminate over, but I do know better than to lie to la policia about handicap parking spots. Like the grooves on an old, scratched record, there I go again... and worse still, I couldn't believe that I was yelling to my wife to hobble! Besides, who even uses a word like hobble anymore?

Hobble: To put a device around the legs of an animal, for example a horse; to hamper, but not prevent movement; a hobbling gait.

What was I thinking? My love for my wife is deeper than anything I've ever known. She has inspired me toward more compassionate relationships with family and more kindness toward animals. I felt small and ridiculous. Hobble? I've always wanted her to be free, to express her true nature, never to hobble. Never wanting to *hamper or prevent her movement.* I was astonished by such a sudden, rapid regression back to an adolescent get-away-with-it-at-all-cost approach to preventing a mordida and saving a few Pesos.

The police truck pulled out of sight. Carol still had no idea why I was yelling at her to hobble. We awkwardly climbed into the van with me feeling very small and very quiet. She looked at me with her palms up, pinching all of her fingers to her thumbs, in the classic Italian sign language of "WTH?"

It was a green flash moment for me.

The path of self-discovery is like seeing the green flash at sunrise, a moment of brilliance, before being washed out by hot glaring sunlight. It can be a glimpse of our true nature.

Today, I am available to see what I need to, to experience who I truly am. My eyes are open. Today, I choose truth and kindness. Today, I look for the green flashes throughout my day.

Sitting on the beach with Carol, the sun hangs above the horizon on the Sea of Cortez. Orange light grows and recedes with the incoming waves along the shore.

I shared my plans for the day with Carol—harvest some veggies from the garden, pick a papaya from the tree, kite surf, do some writing, and maybe take a nap in the hammock…

"Oh, a busy day huh?" she says, "But first, walk with me down the beach to Buena Vista."

As we stand up to walk, two pelicans pass by, gliding low to the water atop the waves. The trailing pelican drafts the lead pelican, mirroring its path with subtle movements of their wings.

On our walk on the beach to Buena Vista we will search for beautiful things, sea glass, driftwood, rounded stones, pieces of tile. But what we find may not be tangible. We might find something more important—inspiration, kindness, freedom, and the wonderment of a green flash—the intangible of living the good life.

The Sea of Cortez
Los Barriles, Baja California Sur, Mexico

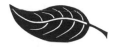

*"With every drop of water you drink, every breath you take,
you're connected to the sea."*

~ Sylvia Earle *(Marine Biologist)*

The turquoise Sea of Cortez summons me even before I
awake. The drubbing sounds of shore break, or the absence
of the sound of waves, visits me in dream. Dry, desert winds
whistling through the palm trees at night tell a story. I think
of the fish resting, or some coming to life at night in a world
just below the surface of my mind.

On wave-less, wind-less days, when there is no surfing
or kite surfing and after a cup of tea in the morning, I
Stand Up Paddle (SUP). I paddle to train for race and endurance events, particularly the Vegan 1 Day seventy-two mile
paddle around Lake Tahoe.

I paddle to feel good, to feel alive, to connect with the
ocean, and let the ocean connect with me.

Stepping onto my SUP, I ride the conveyer belt of life, the liquid life force of planet earth where the abundance of ocean life is all around me, a part of me, and I am a part of it. As a vegan, I'm often asked if I eat fish, and if not, why. For me, the answer is easy, "No, I don't eat fish. I love the ocean, and I don't need to eat fish in order to be healthy." I don't consider fish to be objects, but rather they are social animals, good-natured and curious. I've experienced fish communicating around me using sound, body language, even bubbles. I could never imagine clubbing over the head an animal that I consider to be a friend, an ocean visitor, a fellow swimmer, a surfer, and an earthling just like myself.

In spite of the ongoing damage to the Sea of Cortez ecosystem by over-fishing, it is still one of the most biologically diverse marine habitats on the planet where the feeding, breeding and nursing of some of the world's rarest marine animals takes place.

When paddling, I am a part of the fabric of life. Layered with the tiniest of jellyfish, green phytoplankton, sea turtles, mobula rays, sharks, dorados, dolphins and blue whales (the largest animal on the planet). In fact, the Sea of Cortez is home to the most diverse species of whales anywhere – fin, blue, sperm, Bryde's, humpback, grey, and orca. On the ocean, I am a nonentity in human terms just the way I like it. I am free of identity. I am one among many, salt water our thread of connection.

Being alone on the ocean doesn't scare me, because I never feel alone. I see the ocean as a friendly environment. I float, my board floats, and I am a strong swimmer. I can hold my breath for several minutes at a time. I can also comfortably free dive as deep as sixty feet. And yes, there are creatures in the ocean that, given the right opportunity, would eat me. And the strength of the ocean is far more powerful than I ever will be. But, there are also turtles and dolphins, waves to surf, and whales to visit. My connection with the ocean far outweighs the dangers. Sometimes I feel more comfortable in the ocean than I do on land. I seem to be part fish and I can swim better than I can walk.

In the ocean, if there's a problem I need to deal with it. In other words, if I'm a long way out, and there is an emergency, I need to self-rescue. I need to know how to read the ocean, observe wind lines and direction, recognize currents, follow the weather, and also of importance, to know myself.

I have to ask myself where, and in what circumstance, am I comfortable? And when finding myself out of my comfort zone, I need to stay calm.

Rarely do I paddle with a buddy. I have one or two buddies who could or would paddle with me, but the truth is I don't mind paddling alone. The beauty of the ocean keeps me company. In the absence of a buddy system, I tell or write Carol a note, letting her know where I'm going. She arrives home to notes like.... "9 a.m. went paddling northeast, probably 8 miler. Don't start worrying until siesta time.... check that... don't worry at all".... or "paddling to Ed's, should be a down-winder coming home." Some of it is a foreign language to Carol. It's primarily for Carol to pass the information along to one of my ocean buddies to organize a rescue, if I were long overdue. Although Carol surprises me once in a while with a question peppered with surf lingo like, "How was the up-winder? Catch any good swell on the way home?"

On this particular day, my note to Carol reads: "Going to get wet, home soon." I grab my SUP, paddle, and shoulder hydration pack and do some yoga stretching on the beach. It's 8 a.m. The wind is calm and the sun is warm.

As I paddle straight out from the beach, I pass a sea lion floating on his back. He has been stationed in the same spot in recent days, his front flippers sticking out of the water, as he seems to be sunning himself, or resting. I paddle closer to investigate. Twenty feet away he suddenly notices me, gives off a couple of muffled yelps and dives under. Popping up for air, he looks back over his shoulder wondering where I came from and how I got so close without being noticed sooner.

I remember a time surfing a Northern California wave in Santa Cruz, California. Unbeknownst to me, a sea lion was surfing the same wave underwater until deciding to catch some air right in front of me. We gently hit each other, causing no harm, just knocking each other off the wave. The two of us, distinct species, shared a common space which was more than the wave. It was also each other's safety, and our mutual surprise. Our simultaneous yelp came from the gut.

To surfers like me, sea lions are the big dogs of the ocean. They have a loud bark that gets people's attention, but they are more playful than many cranky, territorial surfers I know. For me, sharing the ocean with playful seals and sea lions is a privilege.

In the distance, on the Sea of Cortez, I see a floating plastic bag and paddle over to pick it up. Plastic bags are a plague to the ocean. On the leeward side of most landfills in Baja, loose plastic bags are as abundant as Saguaro Cactus.

Plastic bags are scars on the Baja landscape and are a camouflaged danger for marine life wreaking havoc on turtles and coral reefs. If I stop at the market in town for nothing more than two avocados, by the time those avocados get to the other side of the cajero (cashier), BAM, an eager, smiling Mexican kid has los aguacates in double-ply plastic bags ready to go!

These ubiquitous plastic bags can easily make the journey from the market into the ocean, and once there they damage coral reefs and kill sea turtles and other marine life. Not accepting the offer of plastic bags in a Baja market elicits a look of curiosity. Sometimes if the market isn't too busy, I use the moment as an educational opportunity, drawing a chart and diagram with my hands in the air... market- plastic bag- wind- cactus- wind- arroyo- rain- ocean- turtle- dead.

The mention of turtles sparks interest because there is a growing connection to turtle conservation throughout Baja, and in fact, all of Mexico. In a ten-mile stretch of beach around my house in Los Barriles, more than 37,000 sea turtle eggs (Leatherhead, Loggerhead, and Green sea turtles) are laid each year. Because of the local Grupo Tortuguero many more of these sea turtle eggs are protected and hatched.

Coming in off the water after a paddle, my surf trunk pockets are usually stuffed full with floating plastic bags I have collected.

The plastic bag I paddle over to retrieve isn't a plastic bag at all. It's a medium size green turtle that duck dives under as I come near. Lately, I've seen fewer plastic bags in the ocean and more sea turtles.

This is a monumental change in a community and culture that used to view the eating of turtle eggs as an aphrodisiac. People in Mexico used to commonly make scrambled eggs for breakfast from turtle eggs. Myths about animal foods are hard to break, especially if they involve male virulence. And yet, education turned the culture around in Mexico. Now, turtle egg nests on the beach are posted and protected. When the baby turtles hatch, it's celebrated as a community event.

The latest destructive trend in animal consumption is the Asian market for shark fin soup, considered a delicacy and irresponsibly used in Traditional Chinese Medicine to boost sexual potency. However, people usually ingest more dangerous levels of mercury from pollution in the shark fins than they do the desired sexual aid.

Most unfortunate are the sharks themselves who, many times, have their fins cut off, and the rest of their bodies are discarded back to the sea while still alive only to die, desperately unable to swim and survive.

Meanwhile, as I dig my paddle into the warm ocean all around me, mobula rays start to jump in a crescendo of dance. As if soaring under the water the rays now breach the surface flying into the air! They ascend two to four feet above the sea, flapping their wings as they fly. Twisting in the air, somersaulting, sometimes landing upside down. It is a swimming and flying display of wild expression.

Some nights in Baja, before going to sleep, the only sounds we hear are the lapping shore-break and the sound of what locals call "popcorn." The sound of thousands of rays breaching and slapping against the surface of the water sounds just like the popping of popcorn. They are the sounds of life from the beating heart of the ocean.

The Sea of Cortez has the largest concentration of mobula rays in the world. And yet the scientists are baffled as to why the rays leap out of the water. Theories include a courtship, or the mobula could be getting rid of parasites, or playing, or by accident—simply running out of water in untamed gesticulations that result in a breach. The wonderful thing about the different theories of their breaching is that we want to know why, but we still don't. The unknown splendor of the lives of ocean beings is still slowly revealing itself to us. One thing for certain is that they sure look happy.

It's a beautiful thing to see my fellow creatures in their element and happy. I know I like being in my element and happy and this is one of the precious gifts we share in common.

Today, below my board, all I see are waves of black soaring wings, and above the surface random disc-shaped flying saucers. Then, with a curious abruptness, the popcorn stops and the rays disappear. I had never seen this before. Gone. In a matter of moments, thousands of them vanished.

Wondering where they went, I scan the horizon of the ocean. A mile or two off to the southeast I notice what looks like a pod of whales heading in my direction. I crouch down, lowering my ear to the board hoping to hear the eerie moans and whining of the Humpback whale song being amplified. I hear no whale song.

Visually what I make out are the pod's breathing rhythm and cadence, which look more like dolphin. Then, it dawns on me. What I'm seeing are tall dorsal fins! They're orcas, otherwise known as killer whales!

Now I know why the rays left so quickly! Judging from where the orcas are, their measured pace and the direction they're moving, it seems as though I'm positioned directly in their path. *Breathe,* I say to myself. They are an apex-predator species on the ocean. Orcas fear nothing and no one. Great white sharks give ground to orcas.

Be cool, the voice in my head says. I am thrilled to see them, but I'm also a little nervous from the uncertainty of never having had an encounter with orcas. I calm myself with the memories of countless friendly encounters with whales, dolphins, and even makos and hammerhead sharks. Besides, I am two miles off shore. There is nowhere to hide.

It is time to breathe and center myself. Just as the orcas are in their environment, so am I. I inhale deeply through my nostrils. The air smells of sea salt and sunshine.

The situation reminds me of a conversation I had with Carol's brother Peter in New York. As mentioned earlier, Carol's family is New York Italian, and I am a California kid.

"Okay Johnny, come over here, listen, this isn't Lake Tahoe," Peter says. "These people here are nuts. These New York cabbies will kill you. You've got to claim your ground. If you're driving, that's your space, you know. It's like you've got to put a force field out around your car. You can't let them push you around."

Alone, two miles out in the Sea of Cortez, I stand on a SUP board with New York cabbies in the shape of orcas on their way. Ocean-board-paddle-me.

I quietly, confidently claim my space and wait. Living in harmony with the ocean also includes projecting a strong, comfortable sense of self. That kind of confidence and ease is recognized and understood by other species as a clear and appreciated boundary. In other words, *I am not food* posturing is done by many species, including me.

There are streaks of patterned black and white spots, windmilling fins arching in and out of the water. Poetic timing to the sound of their breath. Whoosh, whoosh, WHOOSH.

There are about twelve of them. Four or five of them are large adults, several adolescents, and a few small, younger ones, all of them heading directly toward me. As they near, their path takes them directly under my board! They appear as leaves, floating down a river—effortless. The orcas head north. I follow. At their pace, I fall behind quite a distance. Just as suddenly as the "popcorn" rays disappeared, so do the orcas. Gone. I know the orcas will be coming up for air at some point, but something altered their travel and now I realize why.

The orcas resurface, closer to shore, now separated from each other at strategic points. They swarm the frantic group of mobula rays! Evidently, the rays sensed the orcas presence earlier and bolted for the safety of shallower water.

The orcas begin herding and thrashing the rays at different locations. It was as if the orcas had set up stations, some waiting, others herding, while others feed. I paddle for a closer view. As I get closer, it is a wild scene of a free-for-all. The sea lion, which I had surprised a ways back while it was sun bathing, is on the fringe of the melee. I park myself on the fringe, too. If the sea lion, now an opportunist, feels safe enough in his location, then so do I.

If the sea lion moves, then I move, I think to myself.

Balancing on an SUP in the Sea of Cortez on the fringe of a mobula ray bait ball with fifteen-ton killer whales feeding is not everyone's idea of connecting with the ocean. But I was within my own comfort zone.

My desire to connect with the ocean that I love, and my ocean sensibility give me a broader comfort zone than others might have. Everyone has his or her own comfort zone. I know mine. What looks like a big wave to surf for you, might look like a small wave to surf for me, or vice versa. I trust the inner voice that guides me on the ocean as well as on land.

There is, of course, the other extreme. Some people would prefer to see orcas and dolphin put on a show, and do cute tricks at Sea World, or at other captive locations. But many people may not realize the realities of dolphinariums. Instead of swimming up to 100 miles a day in the open ocean, orcas and other dolphin species in these marine parks can only swim endless circles in enclosures that would seem like bathtubs to you and me. Captive orcas and dolphin suffer chronic stress and weakened immune systems, causing them to die earlier than their wild counterparts. Orcas and dolphin navigate by echolocation, but in the tanks the reverberations from their sonar bounce off the walls, driving some of them insane.

Renowned oceanographer Jean-Michel Cousteau compared the keeping of orcas and dolphins in tanks to "a person being blindfolded in a jail cell." Orcas and dolphin in captivity demonstrate a variety of stress-related behavior such as injuring or killing their trainers, injuring themselves by hitting their heads against the sides of the pools, or even taking their own lives by refusing to eat or coming up for air.

I can imagine how I would feel if I were torn from my family and home and forced to perform silly tricks in a jail cell for the rest of my life. How long could I take it before I became aggressive, or refused to eat, or breathe?

For Carol and me, a vegan way of life seeks to exclude, as far as possible and practical, all forms of animal exploitation, including food and entertainment. One point of interest is that Sea World has recently partnered with The Humane Society agreeing to end the breeding of captive orcas for their shows. This means that the remaining orcas at Sea World are the last orcas of their generation to be bred to live in captivity for entertainment. This step forward is a huge accomplishment and is a direct result of the public pressure of people speaking out on their behalf, and also by not supporting their captivity by purchasing a ticket to their shows. It also shows that many people do care. Speaking out on behalf of orcas and dolphins in captivity, or on behalf of sharks exploited for their fins, or on behalf of sea turtles, or picking up trash in the ocean, are some of the small prices I pay to live on this beautiful, blue planet. These actions, put together by many of us, make a difference in the world.

If everyone on the planet went vegan for just 1 DAY, we would save-

- *Approx. 58 orcas, 2000 dolphins, 227 Beluga whales, and 37 porpoise held in captivity globally.*
- *41 dolphins killed per day globally (for food and bait fishing).*
- *43 whales killed per day globally (for food).*

(Sources: Blue Voice, Sea Shepherd)

Here in southern Baja, there are now three swim with dolphin facilities, with another one being built in San Jose Del Cabo. Tourists on vacation want that "amazing" photo of kissing a dolphin in Cabo, but what they don't recognize is, swim with dolphin pools are a kiss of death for the dolphin.

In the wild, there has never been a reported orca attack on a human. While I don't plan on trying to kiss an orca out on the ocean, I feel safe. Watching the orcas feed while standing on a SUP in the ocean is like watching an avalanche from the safety of the ridge top above the massive moving wave of snow. It is an amazing opportunity to see the beauty of nature and also be a part of that beauty.

The orcas' squeaks and squeals in long pitched song and their amazing ocean ability are awe-inspiring. Their ability to communicate with each other is total perfection. I am in awe. And I am a part of this awe.

My thoughts also drift to how we hold animals (of all kinds) in captivity, and how that diminishes our own freedom, and our own happiness. Not everyone needs to paddle straight into an ocean fracas in order to connect with nature.

We can enjoy the beauty of wild orca and wild dolphin by simply swimming in the ocean, sharing the same water space with such beautiful creatures. We can read a book about their lives, or stand on a hillside overlooking the ocean as we scan the horizon for a whale spout as they seasonally migrate up and down the coast. I don't want to live life behind Plexiglas. I want to engage with my surroundings and feel the beauty of being more than just one among many, but one among all.

After the orca feeding frenzy ends and things start to calm down, I see the sea lion maneuver its way through the area looking for some food as the pod of orcas slowly head north. There are no animals *better than* or *less than* in nature, including us. Nature is equal.

For nonhuman animals in nature, choices for survival are limited, unlike us humans who have an abundance of options. Yet many don't see it. I do see a choice. I'm glad I don't have to eat animals in order to survive. I don't need turtle eggs and shark fins for sexual enhancement, or tuna for protein, or salmon for omega-3 fatty acids, or captive dolphin and whales for entertainment.

For me, living vegan not only provides abundant taste and nutrition, it also has lifted the curtain of separation between others and myself. No longer am I separate from anyone else, including ocean beings. I'm no longer at odds with, or need to take anything from, the sea. The sea that surrounds me when I paddle energizes me when I surf and supports my weightless body as I swim. This is enough in and of itself. The oneness I experience with the ocean is freely shared with me and I in turn share it with others; other people, other animals, all of life... all of us.

The entire time I've been following the orcas, I have also felt the desperate circumstance of the beautiful mobula rays. The rays are closer to the shore. Thousands of them are now "shell shocked," not in the least bit concerned with me as I drift above them on my SUP in five feet of water.

The scene of these once joyous creatures touches my heart. The gentleness and compassion displayed by the rays to each other is both heart wrenching and beautiful. They seem to be swimming around each other, softly gliding over each other, gently scanning themselves, feeling the sandy ocean floor with the tips of their wings, as if taking inventory of the trauma and loss of the day.

In recent years, scientists are confirming what I already know. Fish are emotional beings just like other animals. They live social lives, form relationships, and feel pain.

In a New Scientist article entitled, *Animal Minds: Not Just a Pretty Face*, Culum Brown (associate professor at Macquarie University) writes,

> *Most people dismiss fish as dim-witted pea-brains that spend all day swimming around doing...well, nothing.*

Worse still, others believe that, like Dory in the film Finding Nemo, fish have a 3-second memory span and are doomed to perpetually rediscover the joys of their fish tank or goldfish bowl. And as for culture or social engagement – forget it.

Yet this is a great fallacy. Fish are more intelligent than they appear. In many areas, such as memory, their cognitive powers match or exceed those of "higher" vertebrates, including non-human primates. Best of all, given the central place memory plays in intelligence and social structures, fish not only recognize individuals but can also keep track of complex social relationships.

I paddle back home with a thirst and hunger for fresh coconut water and sliced papaya with lime. I look at my watch. It's 1 p.m. I had been following the sea lion, the mobula rays, and the orca family for five hours.

My note to Carol earlier read, "Going to get wet, home soon." For me, when on the Sea of Cortez there is a need for latitude in understanding the definition of the word soon. Carol knows that when she hears the word soon, it could mean a couple of hours or all day. It's like hearing the word mañana in Mexico.

Earlier in the morning, leaping mobula rays surrounded me as I glided on my SUP over thousands of swimming, soaring wings. If their earlier flying leaps into the air were a celebration, I too was celebrating. And if their gentle touching of each other in the shallows due to trauma and loss was a time of mourning, I too was mourning. How could I not? Why would their capacity for grief be any different from my own?

For now, the popcorn sounds of leaping rays have ended and the Sea of Cortez is silent, but the rays will return. The only sounds that remain are that of my paddle in the salt water and the quiet beating heart of the ocean, just below the surface of my mind. Soon I will be home, but in many ways, I am already home.

Shrimp Like Me

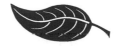

"The most valuable thing we extract from the
ocean is our existence."

~ Sylvia Earle (*Marine Biologist*)

The human condition is such that humans generally seem to learn from first-hand experience. We learn about compassion after receiving it. We learn about health when there is an illness. *DUDE! Don't take the brown acid!* Yes, well, in my life I too have had to learn most things the hard way.

In order to survive on the planet, we need clean air to breathe, clean water to drink and an atmospheric temperature that is not too hot and not too cold in order to maintain earth's climate system.

In one of my very own experiments in living at college and as a newbie to vegetarianism, I survived on marijuana and Doritos. It seems, as though the body says *that crap again, ok fine, I'll make it through another day.* That is, of course, until the body is damaged and there is illness. The body doesn't judge us. The body simply carries on doing the best it can until it can't.

The earth seems no different. War, violence, cruelty... the earth says, *here, have a banana, you must be tired, sit down, take a load off...* No judgment. No exile. No withholding of bananas. The earth is unconditionally supportive of our existence on this planet without contingencies on our behavior—until the earth is damaged and the beauty is destroyed and there is nothing left to eat. Just as our own body has a tipping point for poor health, so does the earth. The earth may not be able to sustain all of our laissez-faire, learn-on-the-fly living.

A question I have is, what will the earth look like in 20 years, 150 years, or 400 years? Will the ocean have any fish left or will the life in the ocean consist of small organisms and jellyfish? It is quite conceivable that a vast majority of the population will eat a vegan or mostly plant-based diet in the future, but will it be by choice? Will it be as a result of earth's depleted resources? Or both?

There is one thing that is certain the facts are unavoidable. Animal agriculture produces 51% of all greenhouse gas emissions. It requires ten times more water, and also ten times more land to produce a meal with meat and dairy than it does to produce the same sized plant-based meal.

It's estimated that most large marine ecosystems will collapse by the year 2048 due to overfishing. Scientists predict large dead areas in the ocean soon if we don't change our ways. We are losing species to extinction in the ocean and on land due to our eating habits and their habitat loss.

After a morning SUP paddle in Los Barriles, Baja, I wondered about what the future on our planet will look like. It was on one of my daily paddles on the Sea of Cortez, that I had just paddled past five shrimp trawling boats after their night of collecting every single living being off the ocean floor that their funnel-shaped nets could hold. Although industrialized fishing is just one of the human activities that threatens the oceans, it is among the most serious.

The shrimp trawlers catch included a very small mako shark, a mobula ray, flounder, hawkfish, puffer fish, eels, starfish, sand dollars, and oh yes, shrimp.

According to a 2014 Oceana report, "Wasted Catch," for every pound of wild shrimp caught, trawlers kill as much as 40 pounds of by-catch. Shrimp trawlers use nets weighted with chains dredging the seabed of all life in its path. It is the maritime version of clear cutting.

Shrimp trawling is comparable to bulldozing an entire section of rainforest to catch a single species of bird. As a result of this form of fishing, the wild shrimp population in the northern Sea of Cortez has virtually collapsed.

It's very odd to hear people describe our community where we live here in Baja as a quaint fishing village. How romantic.

But, there is nothing quaint, nor romantic, about modern day industrial fishing practices.

As I paddled past the shrimp boats, the crew didn't mind my curious perusal of their destructive operations. I went right up to the sides of the boat while standing on my SUP board and made chitchat with the crew. They were more curious about me on my board than why I would be curious of them.

The shrimp boats and their surroundings could be described as floating Superfund sites. The entire surroundings of the boats were a toxic wasteland of destruction. There was the smell of diesel from the oil slick around the boat, floating cigarette butts and empty potato chip bags in the water.

The by-catch of the above mentioned: shark, mobula ray, numerous puffer fish, starfish, eels...floating nearby. Mounds of large Baja shrimp piled onboard.

The crew was four to five men per boat and looked like the results of two-week Meth benders, scary dudes with big eyes looking as though they didn't give a shit about anything. Their look told the entire story. These boys in Baja were doing the best they could to fulfill that vision of depleting the Sea of Cortez by 2048.

According to a 2006 study led by Dr. Boris Worm and a group of international ecologists and economists, three-quarters of the world's ocean are already exploited or depleted and the oceans may be fishless in the near future.

After my paddle, I was standing on the beach next to my neighbor Paul. We looked out at the shrimp boats just off shore from where I had just paddled in. He said to me, "Makes me hungry, looks like we'll be having some shrimp tacos tonight!"

I was dumbfounded. In that moment, the vision of our future hit an all-time low.

Of the seven species of sea turtles living in our oceans, all are listed as endangered or threatened. Every year, more than 50,000 sea turtles are killed from shrimp trawling. The Los Barriles community has a wonderful sea turtle conservation group with wide spread community support. So, the community, including my neighbor Paul, supports the turtles hatching, only to then turn around and support the shrimp trawlers by eating the shrimp, which kills sea turtles.

If people who are living along the coast where these destructive fishing practices take place still support these fishing practices by eating their product, how in the world would the guy living in Bakersfield, removed from the hidden realities of overfishing, make the connection and an informed choice?

My neighbor Paul is a nice person, a kind person. He lends me screwdrivers, vacuum hoses, a generator when there is no power, and has even gently peeled me off the rock seawall after a kite-surfing accident.

So, when my neighbor informed me of his shrimp tacos dinner idea, I did not reflect back to my neighbor the love and support of a friendly universe.

I said, "Look around you man! Try eating veggie tacos once in a while!"

I issued a brief and sharp professor style lecture on the destructive nature of shrimp trawling. I bombarded him with the highest form of my intellect.

"Did you know that industrial fishing accounts for yadda, yadda, yadda...."

My neighbor was not inspired, nor impressed by my plant-based lecture and I felt as small as a southern Sea of Cortez crustacean. This was not one of my finest moments.

My neighbor's lifestyle of remaining comfortably unaware is his choice, but it is not unlike how a lot of people decide to deal with the realities of their food choices. My approach of anger and frustration in communicating to my neighbor was the epitome of being ineffectual, lacking in compassion, and selfish.

The urgency with which my words landed in my neighbor's ear that morning, were motivated by the awareness that we humans seem to be racing to extinction. *No more grouper to eat. No problem. We'll eat tuna. Whoops! Now where'd that one go? No more shrimp in northern Baja? We'll trawl the southern Baja until that collapses. Ugh, there used to be more swordfish, what happened? By the way, anyone see where all of the shark went?*

This tragic demise of sealife will cascade down the fishing line. We seem to be in a race to see who can consume the last tuna, the last marlin, and the last shrimp before they are all gone. *We can't seem to raise our vision beyond the end of our own forks.*

In its hey-day, the Sea of Cortez had some of the largest grouper fish ever seen. Grouper can live up to sixty years and weigh as much as 300 lbs. I've seen a very small grouper on the reef in front of our house, which gave me some hope for their recovery. They are big, lazy, goofy looking fish, quite comfortable being in close proximity to humans. Their curious, friendly disposition worked against them as spear fishermen were able pick them off, one by one, until the population was decimated. They are considered an easy kill. It's like spearing a friendly neighborhood dog.

Some people have a two-dimensional relationship with ocean animals. Either they know how the fish tastes or they wonder if the animal is something they should be afraid of if they're in the ocean. How much can we really understand about an ocean species, its life, behavior, and its value if the only interaction we have with it is with our taste buds?

Dorados are extraordinary swimmers and one of the most beautiful creatures I've ever seen. The dazzling colors of dorados, while alive, go through several hues of golden, blue-green, dark diagonal stripes on each side, and finally fading to a muted yellow-green upon death. How do people know this? Because some people have only seen dorados die, suffering at the end of fishing line and then suffocated on a boat where their brilliant natural colors recede as their life fades out.

It's always a good day on the ocean when I see the athletic brilliance of dorados when I'm kite surfing or SUP paddling. No matter how foolishly hungry people seem, dorados' fundamental value should not be based on the dinner menu.

Dorados play an important role in the eco-system as do shrimp and sharks. Sharks are older than the hills; 450 million years old in fact. They play an enormous role in our oceans. Yet, many people see shrimp and dorados as disposable and sharks as mindless-surfer-eating demons.

Recently, I surfed a hurricane swell at an outer reef a half-mile off shore in Las Barracas, southern Baja. The waves were over-head. I was surfing one of my SUP surfboards and I was the only one out that day, the only human that is. In between set waves, a seven-foot adolescent hammerhead shark would come to the surface and visit me. The shark spent time sixty or so feet away from me just cruising the surface. Then he would get as close as twenty feet where we would do slow, curious, and cautious circles around each other.

Big outside set-waves would come. I would take off to surf them, but the minute there was a lull in the waves, I could count on a shark fin popping back up.

For most people, even surfers, this image conjures up the movie Jaws and evokes fear. Now, I wasn't about to swim over to the shark and give it a tummy rub; had it been a great white shark my experience might have been different. But our encounter was friendly, non-threatening, and intelligent on many levels.

Las Barracas is just on the northern edge of Cabo Pulmo Marine Sanctuary. Cabo Pulmo is one of the most diverse and successful marine sanctuaries in the world. It has a large, healthy population of hammerhead sharks, mostly non-aggressive, as well as many other protected marine species, which is the reason why the surrounding areas of the marine sanctuary like Las Barracas have hammerhead sharks. A protected marine sanctuary means no fishing. A healthy shark population means a healthy marine life population. With no other experiences or knowledge, many people see all sharks in all situations as dangerous man-eaters. People also want to believe that fish can't feel pain, or that shrimp grow like weeds, which of course, is false.

If everyone on the planet went vegan for just 1 DAY, we would save-

- *2,739,726 ocean animals killed per day globally.*
- *27,397 sharks killed per day globally.*
- *178 whales, dolphins and seals killed per day globally.*
- *150 turtles killed per day globally.*

(Source: Oceana 2014 report, "Wasted Catch". Figures include by-catch)

Human unconsciousness with ocean life is as dark and disconnected as the fictional Captain Ahab was in Herman Melville's novel, *Moby Dick*. For some, the sight of an industrial shrimp trawler at sea will evoke a Pavlovian craving response for ceviche tacos. They become blind to the destruction of ocean life below it. However, the human experiment in living off fossil fuels, hamburgers and ceviche tacos seems to be catching up with us. But, while we are confronting the destruction of the oceans, we must also be aware of the struggle to remove the forks from people's salivating mouths.

During that conversation with my neighbor Paul on the beach in Los Barriles, what caught up to me was the net of my own ego. The industrial size opening that constitutes my own mouth and its freakish ability to unleash words. It is the Shakespearean version of clear-cutting the neighborhood.

I am not dissimilar to Paul. I understand the enjoyment of eating seafood. When I was thirteen years old, after a long day of surfing at a spot in Northern Baja called K-38, my family and I ate at a restaurant that served lobster and chile rellenos. The lobster tasted better than anything I could remember eating. The butter was dripping off of the sweet, rich bites of lobster. I kept ordering more.

It was a large family-style restaurant, with the kitchen and stove visible to us all. While waiting for more lobster to be made, I walked up to the kitchen area to watch them prepare the food.

It was there, waiting for more delicious lobster to be prepared that I saw the large red lobsters squirming as the cooks picked them up and dropped them into the boiling water while still alive.

Solemnly I walked back to the dinner table, sad, but mostly feeling disappointed because what I had seen made me lose my appetite. I no longer wanted to eat more delicious lobster that night. It was one of the first connections I made that lobster is an animal, an animal that has a home – the ocean. But they tasted so good.

I wondered how old they were when they were caught, what was their life like in the ocean, how many lobster did the fishermen catch that day, how many were not caught and left in the ocean?

I had so many questions, but all I knew was that I didn't like how I felt about how the lobsters were boiled alive.

I also felt really frustrated by feeling that sadness and confusion because I really wanted to eat more lobster that night.

It would be another four years before I adopted a plant-based diet, but it was experiences like that night that slowly brought me to see what I could do, and wanted to do, for me and the world around me.

There is no such thing as sustainable seafood. Our ocean is being dangerously over-fished with a massive 40% of the fish being fed to chickens, pigs and domestic salmon in factory farming.

Seafood is simply a socially acceptable form of pillaging the ocean. If we plundered all of the birds on land starting with bald eagles until they disappeared. Then we moved on to hawks, seagulls, sparrows, and orioles. Who would be next and who would be safe? The butterfly and hummingbird? Certainly, we couldn't justify bird species' extinction simply because they taste good, could we?

Imagine a world without birds. Now imagine a world without fish. Fish are more valuable to us alive in the ocean than their value is as food.

A functioning ocean filled with life provides the oxygen we breathe, absorbing more CO2 than all forests on land. Every breath we take has passed through the ocean first. An ocean full of life fills us in ways we aren't able to easily quantify.

I imagine if we didn't have life in the ocean, we would quickly understand that loss. On that day, we would know exactly what we are missing – life. Who would we be as a species on a planet where the life around us has vanished? What would we become as we slowly become the vanished, too?

I am not perfect. In fact, I am so imperfect just saying that *I am not perfect* sounds utterly ridiculous. I'm critical, judgmental, often wrong, impulsive, insecure, selfish, irritable, and easily fall into the trap of hopelessness. I am flawed.

I love the idea that *veganism is not a path of perfection; it's a path of kindness.* This concept resonates for me. I care about animals, the environment, and about my relationships with other people.

How I apply the wisdom of those ideals is at times less than ideal.

I offered to my neighbor a heartfelt apology and jokingly asked if he would still consider lending me his 6-foot ladder on occasion. He graciously accepted my amends and joked that the last time I borrowed the ladder it showed back up in his garage with vegan carrot juice stains. I jokingly denied it had anything to do with me.

My neighbor is a good man. Perhaps the beginning point of change is finding the goodness in ourselves and the world around us. And who knows? Maybe a carrot stain on a ladder just may make a difference in opening the eyes of a good man.

If I were able to communicate to ocean beings I would also apologize to them. I would say that I'm sorry for human greed, for our lack of connection, and our short-sightedness. I'm sorry that when I was their only voice on the beach in Los Barriles, I was a petulant surfer, eager to be right, and focused on expressing outrage rather than alternatives to a neighbor.

I am a work in progress. We may or may not already have too much momentum in the wrong direction destroying our oceans beyond recognition, but I want to have hope, be hope and give hope. There is still time to change. We seem to be at a crossroads.

We need to change the industries of killing the ocean into an industry of ocean conservation. I hope we can learn to see beneath the surface of our destructive ways and instead choose life.

I too am learning-on-the-fly. When I am a voice for animals and the ocean, I've learned to ask questions of those I'm speaking with and then to listen to their answers, offering solutions rather than antagonism.

Technically, it's referred to as "having a conversation." Novel idea. They say it works better than lectures. Later that day on the beach with my neighbor, I made a spinach-mango green smoothie to drink and a fried plantain, black bean taco with avocado and cilantro for Paul. Fortunately for all of us there are delicious alternatives to shrimp tacos. I can't say whether or not it changed anything for Paul, but making him a veggie taco changed me for the better.

Regardless of what the future looks like, I know what my here and now looks like. I choose life, compassion, abundance, and love. It is through these undeniable human qualities that I learn to appreciate all of life around me.

I have learned most things in life the hard way, even about love and compassion. I've also grown to discover that an unprocessed, whole-food, plant-based diet feels better than just Doritos and dope. Go figure.

Lupita

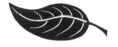

"I would rather make mistakes in kindness and compassion than work miracles in unkindness and hardness."

~ Mother Teresa

During surf trips in Baja, my mind is a steady stream of gratitude. The pleasure of tranquility oozes from my pores. Salt-dried hair and sand stuck between my toes is a testament to my bliss. My equilibrium buzzes as I return home with the energy of the ocean. I am satisfied and satiated with life. But not everything in life is a perfect wave, and the high I get surfing is not the end all.

In Mexico, death is a mask worn by stray dogs and gentle cows. The smell of death arrives unannounced with a sea breeze or with a scent of flowers. Its proximity to us all is more visible in Baja. I am reminded that happiness and grief always share the same road.

Driving, not the surfing, provides most of the adrenaline rushes due to the Aguila—Mexican buses that dominate the narrow shoulder-less road as they rattle the surf boards on top of the car. The main highway is paved while most of other roads off the highway are dirt in what they call washboard, named for the endless bumpy sand rivulets that feel as though they may shake loose engine bolts, gaskets and tooth fillings.

The road to and from Punta Conejo is a washboard. Conejo means rabbit in Spanish. I no longer buy replacement hubcaps because the washboard pulls all the hubcaps off my vehicles and appear as though they're jackrabbits running off the road into the cactus bushes. The turn off the highway to Punta Conejo is at km 80 north of La Paz and is marked with a sign made from what looks like surf stickers and a cactus shrub. The location is officially in the middle of nowhere.

Punta Conejo is a rocky point break and catches lots of swell for surfing. I am a "goofy foot" surfer, standing with my right leg forward. Left breaks allow me to face the wave while surfing, and in Baja, left breaks are less common. Punta Conejo has a beautiful left break when there is a nice south swell.

While driving just south of the Punta Conejo turn off, I see something out of the corner of my eye. I'm not sure I want to see.

I'm feeling stoked from the beauty and power of the ocean. I know that what I think see I out of the corner of my eye will change my emotion. It's one of those moments I'm cognizant that the realm of splendor rubs up against a world of suffering. Shoulder to shoulder, at any given moment, there is sorrow silently standing next to our world of enjoyment.

Reconciling these two worlds has been a path into my own heart. I've never been disappointed by following my heart. My heart compass knows true north.

What I see looks like an injured cow on the side of the road. I have to stop and turn around to know for sure.

Grazing cattle along the roads in Baja is a common sight. The desert landscape provides limited nourishment, while alongside roads wild grass grows provides food. Unfortunately, roads are dangerous places to be for gentle, slow moving cows.

I double back and find a spot off the road. It is indeed a cow, a baby. A car had hit her, but she is still alive. She is lying on her side in a wide ravine and badly hurt.

As I approach, I can feel my body tighten up, cringing in empathy from the agony the calf is experiencing. She wants to move away as I get closer, but can't. I can see the pain and panic in her eyes. Her eyes are those of a child's –helpless and in need.

It appears her front leg is broken, and possibly her back and her jaw as well. I, too, feel helpless. I look around for what I can do and notice her mother standing off in the near distance just far enough to see her, but not too close to the road and me. She is mooing and moaning, calling out to her baby in distress.

I've seen the maternal instincts of many species of animal. But on this day, in the harshness of the Baja heat, with pieces of cactus stuck to her chin from eating scrub brush around cactus, I am deeply moved by the mother cow and her baby's vulnerable predicament.

How long had they been there, I wondered. Tears in my eyes and panic in my chest well up. Surely I was not the first vehicle to have passed by.

I don't know what my options are. It's not like there is a Farm Sanctuary nearby that would come to give care and rescue.

In an odd way, just the mere thought of Farm Sanctuary where farm animals are treated as individuals with love and respect, much like our companion animals (dogs, cats, etc.), adds to my desperation.

The idea of Farm Sanctuary, in itself, is a beautiful one. Farm animal sanctuaries are beacons of hope in a desolate landscape of animal agriculture's brutal treatment of farm animals.

My friend Gene Baur, who is the founder of Farm Sanctuary, comes to mind and I think, *He would know what to do!* He's a dude that could treat a calf's broken leg and give a speech to the United Nations at the same time.

I scan the horizon again, searching for something that I already know is not there. No phones. No Farm Sanctuaries. No Gene Baur. We are alone – a baby, her mother, and me.

I crouch down and stroke the baby's head and neck knowing that she will probably die from her injuries. The least I can do is to stay with her in prayer, or sadness, or companionship as she passes.

Just then, a truck with a trailer pulls up. It stops right in the middle of the road with hazard lights on and three Mexican cowboys meander out of the truck as if on a Sunday stroll. For a brief moment, I feel relief. Yes! There are others and certainly they will help.

But my hopes quickly vanish as they joke and whistle their way over to the scene. To them, this is not a baby in need of help; it is an item to pick up and bring back to the ranch. The careless disregard for a living, feeling being I begin to witness is beyond belief.

They yank on her tail to see if she would stand up. She toppled over on to her head. They tie up her broken legs and pull her up the small ravine by her tail and broken legs. They winch her onto the trailer as her head and body bang on rocks and across the ground.

This is rural Mexico. There are no laws I know of that protect animals of any kind, much less injured calves. The men are blatantly indifferent to the calf's suffering. Indeed, they are causing more pain.

I compel them at every opportunity to stop and change their approach, to recognize the distress of the calf. I am met with disinterest and contempt. "No pasa nada..." (Don't worry, nothing's wrong), they would say. I plead with them to look into the calf's eyes to see her pain and distress as I kneel down facing the calf. This was when they get machismo with me, telling me to, "pasa un lado o sera el proximo" (step aside, or you'll be next).

I know that there was nothing else that can be done. I am as helpless as the calf's mother standing in the distance sharing a broken heart.

In my lifetime, I've been called just about every derogatory, emasculating name there is. Kindness toward animals, especially farm animals threatens people, or at the very least makes them nervous and uncomfortable. Showing vulnerability and care to an animal that to them is nothing more than something to eat challenges their reality. Acknowledging that animals are *someone*, instead of *something*, shakes the whole enchilada of what's for dinner.

But on this occasion, it was the first time in the Spanish language that I was called the familiar, uncreative, unoriginal, derogatory, emasculating names that are used toward men. Sticks and stones may break my bones but words will never hurt me. But these cowboys were quickly preparing to alter their course of action with me by abandoning the name calling shtick for the alternative.

I never returned their angry words. I know these people... these cowboys. They are everyday people you would meet down here in Baja. Good people, the kind of people that give you a firm handshake and look you straight in the eye.

I remember visiting the house of a man named Chuy, who had done some carpentry work on my house in Los Barriles. Chuy is one of the friendliest, easy-going people you could meet. I would never see Chuy without a smile, and on Saturdays, for a half-day of work, he would bring his twelve-year old son to the job to help him.

A very nice man, but at his house, he's running a cock fighting operation.

Yes, cock fighting... the shadowy entertainment, which is understood to be cruel and barbaric to roosters. It is illegal in the USA, but it is being run in the backyard at Chuy's house in Baja, Mexico unencumbered.

All animals, including farm animals, experience joy and suffering, just like you and I... and our dogs and cats, whales, birds, cows, monkeys, chickens and every other creature that breathes and has a pulsating heart.

It's a heavy thought for a Baja cowboy to see animals as living, feeling individuals. These muchachos have jobs to do. Cruelty to animals is taught. Their fathers taught them, who in turn, taught their children, and so on. Children naturally have compassion for animals, but it's been "taught" out of them. Or shamed out of them. Or ignored out of them.

They need to bring their "property" back to the ranch to be "processed." Their macho front is a form of survival in a culture where caring for a crippled calf is for little girls. To them, I have been dropped from another planet, proclaiming "War Is Over, if you want it"... while in bed with Yoko Ono. It's not part of their world.

If everyone on the planet went vegan for just 1 DAY, we would save-

- *5,753 veal calves (baby male cows) killed per day globally (veal is a by-product of the dairy industry).*
- *32,876 lambs (baby sheep) killed per day globally.*

(Sources: United Poultry Campaign, Free From Harm, Occupy For Animals)

As I gather myself, and clear away the tears in order to be able to drive, I think of a woman named Lupita who was a babysitter for my brother, sister and me while growing up in Southern California. She was wonderful, kind, caring and fun.

Lupita came from a very small town along the border south of Tucson, Arizona. I remember my disbelief in hearing about the hardships of her life, including how one of her adult sons drowned in a river he was crossing. He didn't know how to swim, which in itself was inconceivable to me. Why or how was he trying to cross a river while not knowing how to swim?

Also, the fact that he died while Lupita was in the United States away from her family and not having the legal nor financial means of returning to Mexico and then back to USA was heart breaking to consider. The depth and loneliness of such grief is beyond what I can imagine. Living in Baja, I often think of Lupita and see her in the gentle, resilient nature of the Mexican people. Being around Lupita was a soft place.

In my life, it has been the kindness of people like Lupita who have unknowingly been helping me reconcile the world of sorrow with the world of joy. Happiness mixes with melancholy. Nothing is permanent in life, not the waves I surf, the lives of my loved ones, the joy I feel from the ocean, nor the sadness from the world's lack of empathy for animals. I have deep gratitude for the energy of ocean waves, animals for their gentleness, women for their resilient hearts, and also my awareness of the fragility of life.

I've taken to calling the little injured calf on the side of the road Lupita. Little Guadalupe. The last I see of little Lupita, the poor injured baby calf, she is tied up and crumpled against the sidewall in the back of the trailer heading north. Lupita and I shared the unbearable pain of a world that could be so different. As the truck and trailer unsympathetically bounces away up the highway, the heartbreak is left on the side of the road with the calf's mother and me.

I could not stop Lupita's tortured life and tragic end. Neither could I turn away, driving home from a surf trip in her time of need, clutching to the illusion of a surfer's high at the expense of compassion. It was my need to stop...to try. In our brief moment together, perhaps she felt my compassion... my pain for her... my pain for us.

Who stops for the brokenness of another? What price does compassion exact? Living a full life includes the collection of fragments and sorrow that are scattered across the landscape of all of life. To turn away from the sufferer, no matter whom that may be or what form of life that creature has taken, creates a turning away of myself. Who would I become if I were to ignore the vulnerable self on the side of the road? We may bury suffering or mask it in sanitized secrecy behind shielded walls of factory farms or on a desolate landscape of the Baja desert, but it is impossible to truly ignore the consequences of our actions or inaction. On some level, on every level, who we are and what we choose to do is unavoidable. We are altered and shaped by what we do... and what we don't do. I had to stop for Lupita. I had to stop for me.

Lupita shapes me. And for one brief moment, my deepest hope is that my caress of Lupita shaped her. My prayer for Lupita as I drive away is that she feels the love of her mother and the kindness of my failed intervention. And, in some small way, I hope that love helps her on her journey onward, into the great unknown.

Big Blue

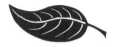

"The mind wants to give up way before the body."

~ Unknown

More than anything else, our minds are the biggest obstacle we will encounter when overcoming a challenge, and as I look at Lake Tahoe I think of the words of my friends who refer to Lake Tahoe as "Big Blue"... really Big Blue! While Carol and I gaze at the moon, I reflect on the confidence-building notion that this will be my eighth SUP journey around Big Blue, but the only thing that my mind wants to see is a HUGE lake! Seventy-two miles, solo, non-stop, paddling at night and most of the next day, every year my mind tells me that I can't do it. It says, *take a short cut, take a nap, hide in the bushes, sleep at a friend's house, or drink a cup of tea, anything other than paddle Big Blue in one day!*

Even though it's the middle of summer, the night air in Lake Tahoe is cold and the water temperature is even colder. The notion to SUP the entire lake alone, in one day, may seem like a crazy idea. In and of itself it is a crazy idea. One person, alone, circumnavigating a 72-mile lake. But this act is not based in and of itself. It is a commitment to a higher cause, a purpose with passion, the very core of my being. It is based on my un-yielding belief that life is created and sustained by our highest selves and our highest ideals.

Yes, someone on the shore would look out at me and think that is a crazy guy who wants attention and publicity. But if they knew that every stroke of the cold blue water beneath my board was a testament to eating and living a compassionate life, that every inch forward was my belief that all life matters and that to round this massive lake in one day is my voice—that eating vegan one day, living to the fullest one day, is a purpose beyond me that lies within me. Then maybe they would understand.

I am not starting a movement for veganism. The movement is here and growing. I am making a statement of who I am and what is important to me, and what I believe is important, vitally important, to the world we live in.

What can one "crazy" person do paddling a board alone in waning night on Lake Tahoe? Everything. To live in the fullness of life is to live the essence of life. No matter who will listen or not listen. No matter what people think. No matter what. Life has given everything to me and living a plant-based life is an integral part of my spirit.

The genesis of the idea evolved as Carol and I set out to raise money for the work of Farm Sanctuary, after an inspired meeting with its co-founder, Gene Baur. Farm Sanctuary's mission is to protect farm animals from cruelty, inspire change in the way society views and treats farm animals, and promote compassionate vegan living.

Carol and I have both adhered to a plant-based diet for over 30 years, working on campaigns for the protection of whales in the world's oceans and of wildlife on land. But, it was the meeting with Gene in 2008 that inspired us to focus our individual resources on raising money for Farm Sanctuary's work. After three years, and paddling three circumnavigations around Lake Tahoe at a more casual pace, stopping overnight to camp, and enjoying delicious vegan food prepared by Carol along the way, our project raised over $11,000.

But I needed more of a challenge and we both saw that people in general needed to challenge themselves to do more as well. It's easy to give money; it's harder to change our habits. (No one supports animal cruelty, yet most people eat animals). Animals endure brutality in animal agriculture beyond our wildest imaginations.

Of equal significance is the fact that climate change may be the greatest existential threat to all species on earth, and yet many people are unaware that animal agriculture contributes more greenhouse gas emissions than any other industry. Most people's expectation is that someone else, or our political system should (or will) do something to change the dire realities of such dramatic damage to our environment. Yet somehow, the individual is seemingly left out of the equation, and what remains is societal inaction.

While the public generously contributes donations that fund Farm Sanctuary's vital work, people seem to lack fundamental connections to why, and how, each of us can make a difference in the world through our own food choices. The Vegan 1 Day project was born to amplify that notion.

I will SUP non-stop the entirety of Lake Tahoe in one day, and in place of financial contributions to Farm Sanctuary, people will pledge their personal investment to adopt a vegan diet for at least one day. One day out of the year, one day a month, one day a week, or one day at a time. Go vegan 1 day, maybe one day you'll go vegan! The choice becomes yours.

Holding hands, Carol and I walk down the moonlit path to the lake with my SUP board and paddle. It's 3 a.m. and the wind is calm.

I prepare my mind for all the *expected* obstacles—leg cramps, stomach cramps, serenity, hunger, fatigue, boredom, elation, and the list goes on.

I also prepare my mind for the *unexpected*—the full moon to hide behind clouds, making navigation almost impossible, and other variables not yet considered. Last year, wind direction changed, pushing nearby wildfire smoke from the east into the area, as I coughed and squinted my way around the lake using the shoreline like a blind man reading Braille.

Carrying the board and paddle, as we get closer to the lake, we see the shimmering moonlight on the water. The calmness of Carol's voice soothes me, "It's so beautiful," she says.

Every year, it's the same scenario, I look at the lake, and feel overwhelmed. But one of those little miracles happens when I actually put the board in the water and stand on it. I feel the motion with the paddle and I relax and sink into enjoying the moment. I see the beauty of my surroundings and I realize that it's an adventure!

Will I make it around the lake? Who knows and who cares? I put the blade of the paddle into the water, pulling on the paddle, stroke after stroke, as I check out my paddle technique. I look around to notice the stunning, pristine beauty of Lake Tahoe, and feel the gratitude of the gift it is to be alive, and I am catapulted instantly into the moment, the greatest miracle of all, where I have energy and I feel hopeful.

Inevitably, I will again start thinking about the finish and gently remind myself to stay in the moment. I chuckle at my mind's coy ability to distract, again noticing the details of my surroundings, bringing myself back to the moment, and so it goes, seventy-two miles around Lake Tahoe, one beautiful, miraculous moment at a time.

The process I go through paddling around the lake is quite similar to the external challenges that many people experience going vegan. For the person new to a plant-based diet, there will be the metaphorical challenges of navigating wildfire smoke-filled skies, head winds, or rough waves; but, for me, while paddling Lake Tahoe, my resistance to an obstacle can be far worse than the actual obstacle itself.

Most people, like myself have a very difficult time watching animal abuse. If the abuse farm animals endure is so bad that we can't even watch it, is it something we should be willing to support when we sit down to eat?

The answer for me is no. These animals are abused because we pay to abuse them when we buy meat, dairy, and egg products.

When I explain how going vegan is a viable solution, and choosing to eat plants instead of animals is a simple yet effective alternative to the inherent cruelties of the meat industry, blah blah blah, all they can see in their mind's eye (with an overwhelmed look on their face) is their Big Blue. Will it be an adventure, exploring new, healthier foods? Nope. Most people see a large obstacle, in the shape of Lake Tahoe, where they will toil in boredom and deprivation, paddling in perpetuity, while eating cardboard and grass clippings. *En el contrario!* A life caring about others, the environment, and our health, while eating delicious vegan food is hardly a life of deprivation.

But because of our habituation to animal foods, you will have a difficult time telling that to someone standing on the shore, contemplating the great vegan crossing. In fact, it's much like how I feel as a SUP paddler standing on the shore looking at the enormity of circumnavigating Lake Tahoe.

Everything we want to accomplish in life takes intentionality. Whether we're adopting a plant-based diet or we want to paddle around Lake Tahoe, the intention behind our actions helps shape our experience. For me, the paddle around the lake is a spiritual journey, a pilgrimage I take every year. I am healthy and grateful to be alive. Paddling seventy-two miles around the lake under a full moon is a beautiful thing to do. For me, living vegan transcends my ordinary self and sanctifies my soul. It's my passion for living my core value that all life matters, and that the enjoyment of that life is something to be experienced and shared. My intention is to do something good while living the fullness of one day.

In order to paddle Lake Tahoe in one day (less than 24 hours), I paddle at night, as well as all day. Using a head-lamp while paddling illuminates only a small area around me, and because of the arm stroke motion of paddling, combined with the issue of balancing while standing on a SUP board with just a headlamp, I am completely disoriented.

Paddling under a full moon on Lake Tahoe illuminates features of the shoreline well enough to navigate. The full moon is also a symbol of our collective awakening—a prayer for animals suffering in the meat industry and our hope for a more compassionate world.

Carol and I stand next to each other, arms around each other, looking at the moon as if waiting for inspiration to write a poem. She whispers in my ear, "You can do it. Go get 'em Johnny."

Her kiss feels like nourishment. It will be her voice I hear when I'm miles from home and the demons of doubt and negativity come for a visit. I can count on the appearances of the hideous four horsemen of fatigue, loneliness, frustration and despair. Overly dramatic? Maybe, maybe not.

I will feel one or all of these more than once, and a thought of Carol will help, or a shot of green juice made with kale, celery, mango, watermelon, maca, and spirulina from my hydration pack, or a glance up at the moon and sky.

On the shore of Lake Tahoe, Carol and I say a prayer for spiritual protection and strength. I enter the cold, calm waters with the companionship of the full moon, my thoughts of Carol and our hope for a more compassionate world for animals.

As I push away from the shore, I am aware of being a small person on a large lake. The clanking of a buoyed sailboat mast, my paddle bumping against my board, the increasing sounds of my breath builds in my field of awareness. The sounds of the night on the lake are amplified, but the type and the direction from where the sounds come can be confusing. It feels as though my ears are as large and sensitive as the California mule deer that Carol and I see on the hillside around our home.

Every sound, and the direction from where the sound comes, is registered and analyzed. I listen for the lapping water around unseen hazardous rocks, or worse, a rogue motorboat full of partiers or fishermen. A serene 3 a.m. full moon paddle can very quickly become a game of Marco Polo with a drunk boater.

Even though I've been clean and sober now for many years, the world of alcoholism seems to follow me around like a stray dog in Mexico. In fact, there is a house on the lake in Incline Village that no matter the time of night there is a party going on. I paddle past the Incline Village party house; whether it is 10 p.m., or 3 a.m., all one can hear is bad music and loud people. I can hear the drunken conversations for miles even after passing that house.

It's an interesting paradox. I stand upright on a slick, beautifully crafted SUP, holding a long paddle, on the calm, unspoiled waters of Lake Tahoe; the lake so still it mirrors the night sky, with the full moon lighting my way like a scene out of a Disney movie. Yet, from along the shoreline, drunken rave music blasts out into the wildness sounding like a scared, confused hyena being chased by an angry bear. It's an opportunity for me to remember from where I came without judgment, but with deep gratitude that that existence no longer is a life-destroying part of me. That used to be me, but things have changed. Getting sober will do that. Now I'm a dreamer, standing on a SUP board, paddling around a lake in the middle of the night.

I'm reminded of a couple of neighbors of ours in Baja, Mexico. Phil and Sandy were old, sweet, but hard drinking ex-pats. Sound also carries in Baja. Due to the fact that we're always outside, the neighborhood hears most outdoor activity and conversations.

Phil and I became good friends over the years before he died. He knew about my love of flying and my being a paragliding pilot. We would talk about his collection of vintage remote controlled airplanes he built by hand. Some of the airplanes seemed large enough for a person to fly. He would sit on his outside patio in the mornings, while building RC airplanes, and sing beautiful, deep-voiced acapella versions of Frank Sinatra recordings, filling the neighborhood with song.

But when the drinking started in the evenings, it could turn a corner, so to speak. It could go one of two ways, Dr. Jekyll or Mr. Hyde. There was less uptown Frank Sinatra and more downtown Frank Sinatra.

I related to Phil. My drinking and drug use created a deeper, darker hole in my soul, taking me further and further away from my heart and my dreams. Awakening to that reality is why I'm sober today.

On the lake, my paddle stroke is strong, but relaxed, the Incline Village party house sounds fade, the full moon, in and out of clouds, as I approach Chimney Beach on the east shore. I smell cedar, charcoal remnants from a campfire. In the water, my paddle makes the sound of a trickling brook. I avoid the incidental taps from my paddle against my board so as not to interrupt the cool water sounds broken by the intermittent quietness between strokes. I sip from my hydration pack of green juice with spirulina and maca and eat a few bites of an apple-cherry-and-oats energy bar. Although I'm not hungry, it's important that I keep adding nutrient-dense, energy-sustaining vegan foods a little at a time all the way around the lake so I avoid nausea and cramping.

So, what is a vegan (and veganism) you might ask? I like the definition used by the Vegan Society. "Veganism is a way of living, which seeks to exclude, as far as possible and practicable, all forms of exploitation of, and cruelty to animals for food, clothing, or any other purpose." For me, this *do less harm* philosophy is easy to follow. If there is an alternative to cruelty, why not choose it?

We humans think of ourselves as an exceptional species on this planet; that we have the most intelligence, with the most sophisticated culture, and are the most spiritually relevant. Yet, humans have caused more destruction on the planet than any other species, and we are, by far, the most brutal. Human violence is a scourge on the planet and animals have paid a heavy price for living amongst us.

We want to believe that farm animals live a beautiful life on green pastures before willingly laying down their lives for the sustenance of mankind. Nothing could be further from the truth. The vast majority of animal suffering happens in the food industry. Slaughterhouses are arguably some of the most violent places on earth. Out of sight, out of mind.

In the United States, every twelve seconds, a farm animal is slaughtered. Most are killed by either having their throat cut or a chest stick inserted cutting close to the heart, both resulting in the animal bleeding to death. Animal agriculture is industrialized violence, where some animals spend most of their lives in small cages, unable to stand up or move around.

In the book, *Why We Love Dogs, Eat Pigs, and Wear Cows*, psychologist Melanie Joy explores why people are disgusted by the thought of eating a golden retriever, but happily enjoy beef, chicken, pork and seafood.

The belief system that eating animals is *normal, natural, and necessary* keeps animal suffering largely out of people's awareness.

It seems as though the reason why people eat animals is because people eat animals. Wait, what? In other words, the reason why most people eat animals is because.... most people eat animals. People do what other people do.

And to be fair, it's not just the herd mentality at work. The propaganda machine of the meat industry uses brilliant, yet deceptive ad campaigns to put a happy face on products that cause bad health, harm to the environment, and suffering to animals. The industry also uses legislation to try to keep the public from seeing the harm it causes with so-called Ag-Gag laws, where the filming of animal cruelty, not the cruelty itself, is a crime. As a result, the consumers keep consuming, leaving little opportunity to question why we eat what we eat.

Paddling alone, my mind wanders; a small wave rocks my board. Squinting in the darkness, I stop paddling and instantly go into high alert for a night boater. I'm within twenty feet of shore with huge boulders all around me. These massive boulders were left by melting glaciers from Desolation wilderness. As the snow retreated to higher ground, it left in its place a Zen rock garden underwater and on the shore.

No need for concern, I'm protected by the rocks and the small wave that hit my board is rogue. There are no boats within sight. I take the opportunity to relax for a moment and chug some green smoothie made from avocado, spinach, maca and spirulina, which I've brought with me for sustenance. I see the outline of Cave Rock in the distance and continue paddling.

As a child, I was raised on meat, dairy and eggs. I loved pork chops and applesauce, lobster and butter, grilled cheese and bologna sandwiches. It was only when I questioned eating animals thirty-three years ago that led me to vegetarianism, then veganism.

When I was sixteen years old, I had a friend who worked in the shipping department at the Farmer John pig processing plant in Los Angeles, California. I needed a job and I asked him if he would help set up a job interview for me. He agreed and explained what the work was like in the loading and shipping department, but he also described the pig processing work environment as well. As he described the pig slaughter process, from the beginning to the end, I couldn't believe it.

The hooks, and the bleeding to death, and the sounds of squealing pigs still alive while being dismembered... I was shocked. I had no idea such places existed. I'm not sure how I thought ham and bacon ended up on my dinner plate, but in my wildest fantasies I would never have imagined how brutal and barbaric slaughterhouses were. I was having a difficult time reconciling how and why such places needed to exist in the world. To be honest, I felt worse for the people who had to work in that environment than I did for the animals, and in an instant I changed my mind about wanting to work there. It would still be another year before I went vegetarian.

With each paddle stroke on Lake Tahoe, I focus on my paddle technique. The more efficient I am now, the more energy I conserve for later. The soothing, meditative focus on paddle technique brings me into the moment, where it's easy to breathe and I relax. The lake elevation is 6,200 feet, less oxygen to breathe, but closer to the moon and stars. Just below the full moon, there is a bright star that I hadn't yet noticed. I carry with me while paddling water, green juice and green smoothie in separate hydration packs, homemade energy bars and a portion of lentil loaf. All vegan. All nutrient dense. All delicious. The taste of the energy bars is rich and filling, and I draw on my hydration pack, enjoying the view of the moon, and his new little buddy, the bright star.

There is a myth that a life without animal foods is a life prone to malnutrition and deprivation. Good taste is the first thing people notice and comment on when eating the vegan foods Carol and I prepare. A whole-food plant-based diet is full of taste, nutrition and satisfaction. Once I started to explore the world of plants, a diverse array of taste opened up to me. According to the Encyclopedia of Life Support Systems (EOLSS), studied by the United Nations Educational, Scientific, and Cultural Organization (UNESCO), the earth has more than 80,000 species of edible plants. As a vegan, I eat a vast variety of whole, plant-based foods.

The green smoothie I drink balancing on my SUP, made from spinach, avocado, maca and spirulina, is a blend high in nutrition with fatty acids and lots of protein. I can almost feel a kick of energy with mental clarity and emotional stability as it digests.

Going vegan excludes only three things: meat, dairy and eggs. It happens that those three things (meat, dairy and eggs) are in virtually every prepared food and at every meal for most people. In one of my green smoothies, I get more nutrition from phytonutrients, vitamins, fiber, healthy fats, chlorophyll, and live-food enzymes than many people get all week.

Protein? Yes. Plants. Plenty. There is more protein in a serving of our curried lentil loaf than there is in a serving of beef. Thirty-six grams of protein to be exact, in a healthy-size serving of lentils, compared to 32 grams in the same serving size of beef. And how does plant-based nutrition taste? Off the hook! Remember, there is a diversity of 80,000 edible plant source foods on the planet.

As I paddle the entirety of Lake Tahoe for the Vegan 1 Day project, I think of our human potential and how we can dream a better dream for our world. Better health, less violence, less cruelty to animals. I reach with my paddle, churning the water eddying past my board as I settle into a comfortable rhythm. The night air is cool and the stillness of the lake relaxes my mind.

As I paddle past Cave Rock, I have been on the lake for three hours. The full moon is descending behind the west side of the crest of the Sierra Nevada Mountains, and to the east, there is the first sign of sunlight above Spooner Summit. There have been no drunken speedboaters to worry about, and since the party house in Incline Village, no human sounds. The only sounds I hear are coyotes yapping in the hills and California gulls and grebes on the water swimming out of my oncoming path.

The California gulls of the Sierra are pristine white and shine on the lake under the full moon. The eared grebes migrate this time of year, probably ending up at Pyramid Lake. The grebes are diving, duck-like birds that spend their entire lives on the water. Enjoying the moment, I sit on my board. I am alive, fully alive. I absorb every sound, feel the board beneath me and the lake that holds me in the night air. To be here, to be now, is the greatest gift this journey has to offer. I drink from my hydration pack, and eat a homemade energy bar, made with dates, almonds, oats, pecans, peanut butter and coconut oil. I feel the food with every bite. I swallow the richness of its life-giving sustenance that calls me back to why I'm here in the first place. I am here to celebrate that I am here.

The energy fills me, but the moment fulfills me. I can no more separate what goes into my body from what surrounds my body. The mountains, the moonlit silk water that cradles and gently rocks me, the coyotes howling in the distance, the birds and fish have all invited me into their world. And I have invited them into mine. We spend this miraculous moment as equals. Not just as one among equals, but as equally one.

This is why I live the way I live, make the choices I make, do what I do to bring life to life rather than take life. Life is too precious to destroy in any way shape or manner. This moment, this small moment becomes the compilation of all moments. And I am full...fully alive.

I can see the lights of the casinos in South Lake Tahoe and stand up to continue paddling. It does not break the miraculous moment. It simply changes it into the next moment. I go from the wilderness of Cave Rock to the wilds of South Lake.

The slowest portion of the paddle, in darkness, is behind me. A 4-5 mph side/head wind develops from the southeast. It's now time to increase my paddle stroke cadence before stronger winds develop later in the day. An hour later, arriving in South Shore, the wind changes direction and now comes out of the northwest. Of course! It was a head wind while going south, and now a head wind while going west. While the afternoon west winds (8-12 mph) in the summer called the Zephyr winds are fairly predictable, the other variable winds from random directions throughout the day are nonsensical. I plan the entire paddle around having the Zephyr winds at my back for the last leg of the paddle, but the other random, unpredictable winds are crazy making. Trying to figure them out while paddling is a physical and mental drain. If I think too long about them, I will fall into a negativity trap of frustration and anxiety. I put my head down, paddle, and smile.

I arrive at Emerald Bay at about 9 a.m. It's beautiful. The color of the sky is pale blue and the color of the lake is deep blue. No wind! There are some tourist boats starting to come into the bay; a couple with a dog in a kayak wave to me. I feel good. I feel really good, too good for having just paddled over thirty-five miles! I look over my right shoulder at the other side of the lake from which I came. Crystal Bay, where I last saw Carol hours ago, is barely visible. It looks like a long, long way home! I wonder if I will make it. I can't imagine NOT making it. Am I feeling some sort of natural high that will soon lead to a crash?

Emerald Bay is the jewel of Tahoe. It's virtually enclosed by mountains all around, the Sierra crest and Desolation wildness to the west, with a small opening connecting the bay with the rest of Tahoe. On the far western end of Emerald Bay there is a small island with a small Scandinavian style rock structure used many years ago as a teahouse by the family that lived in Vikingsholm.

I paddle around the Emerald Bay Island once, which takes all of five minutes. And then I do another five-minute lap around the island. It's a victory lap of sorts. I'm feeling good, so why not? Enjoy the day, twice around the halfway point! Just as I complete the second lap around the island, a 4 mph head wind comes up out of the east. Ha! I feel so good that no obstacles in my path can deter me. I paddle out of Emerald Bay, where the wind lets up. Half an hour later, as I begin the last leg of the journey along the west shore, as if right on cue, I feel tired and overwhelmed.

I've run out of green juice from my hydration pack so I filter fresh drinking water out of the lake. I eat a square of a banana and almond butter sandwich on sprouted grain bread. I drink the last of my spinach smoothie. I get a bump of energy and paddle onward down the west shore. I think of Carol at home, maybe sipping tea, or thinking good thoughts, and I feel hopeful. I feel fortunate to have a local community of people, including Carol, who care about animals and the environment. I am alone on the lake, but Carol and I are not the only people in our community who carry a message of compassion for animals.

Like myself, others have completed endurance challenges to promote the Vegan 1 Day message. Monica Quinones, Rob Gorder, Billy Howard, Tom Kalange, Heidi Timinsky, Ryan Peterson, David Robertshaw, Kim Kerrigan, Travis Weaver, Alida Labia, Yolanda Labia, and Gary Talbot have run or biked separate endurance events or paddled portions of the lake with me. Although for the last five years I've paddled the lake alone, the Vegan 1 Day community and its message of helping others adopt a vegan diet accompanies me and motivates me when I am tired and overwhelmed.

If everyone on the planet went vegan for just 1 DAY, we would save-

- *100 billion gallons of water per day, enough to supply all the homes in New England for 4 months*
- *1.5 billion pounds of crops per day otherwise fed to livestock, enough to feed the state of New Mexico for more than a year.*

- *70 million gallons of gas per day, enough to fuel all the cars of Canada and Mexico combined with plenty to spare.*
- *3 million acres of land per day, an area more than twice the size of Delaware.*
- *33 tons of antibiotics per day.*
- *2 billion animals killed per day (land and sea)*

And if everyone, just in USA went vegan for just 1 DAY, the U.S. would prevent-

- *Greenhouse gas emissions per day equivalent to 1.2 million tons of CO2, as much as is produced by all of France in a single day.*
- *3 million tons of soil erosion per day, $70 million in resulting economic damages.*
- *4.5 million tons of animal excrement per day.*
- *Almost 7 tons of ammonia emissions per day, a major air pollutant.*
- *20 million animals killed per day (land and sea).*

> *(Sources: "Livestock's Long Shadow" (United Nations), the World Bank, and calculations of Noam Mohr, a physicist at the Polytechnic Institute of New York University.)*

One-day matters, our food choices each and every day matter. One of the most helpful concepts I've learned from living sober is to live one day at a time, taking each day as it comes. This mind-set allows me the freedom to not get overwhelmed and discouraged by imagining how difficult it would be to keep my resolutions for the rest of my life. I take it day by day.

As early as high school, I was a full-blown addict/ alcoholic. My nickname was *Mellowfield*. Drop the Merry from my last name Merryfield, insert Mellow, smoke some dope, and bingo, you've got Johnny Mellowfield. I was like Bjorn Borg as a tennis player, seemingly without any emotion. Whether winning or losing at Wimbledon no one would know. I may have had the genetic tendency for alcoholism, but the reality is that I buried myself away from my feelings. I was self-medicating my feelings of sadness, depression, trauma and insecurity. Getting sober for me was like having all of the lights come on in the room. I got all of my feelings back at the same time. Now imagine John McEnroe at Wimbledon after a controversial line call. That was me, a little more, shall we say, emotionally volatile.

Before getting sober, I was having small moments of awakening. I can remember Thanksgiving 1983, just before I turned eighteen; my aunt and my mother were preparing a turkey for us to eat. All I wanted to do was to eat some food and leave the house to get high. They both stood over the oven, rubbing butter on the flesh colored skin of the large bellied turkey and lifting the headless bird up by her arms. It reminded of how someone would lift a human baby out of the crib. The image startled me. I was hung over from the day before, but not hallucinating on drugs. I looked again at my mother and aunt preparing the turkey in the roasting pan, as they shoved the undercarriage full of stuffing. The bird looked more like a dog lying on his or her back, waiting for a tummy rub, but mangled and deformed. Needless to say, the turkey looked more like a helpless animal and less like dinner. I was irritated, felt trapped by a loving family, and heartsick from an un-welcome vision of death.

Of course I had some of the more conventional epiphanies as well, such as when my younger brother Jim was standing over me as I took a drunken nap in the bathroom, head resting on the toilet, sick and immobile from another day in the life. My brother's question, *"What the f*ck are you doing with your life?"* didn't exactly require a response, even if I could muster one.

When getting sober, I had no idea who I was, or how to deal with feelings. Early in sobriety I would hear that there is some good news and there is some bad news about living sober. The good news is, you get your feelings back, and the bad news is, you get your feelings back. Bjorn Borg meets John McEnroe. The thawing of the heart and mind in sobriety isn't pretty, but as they say, welcome to humanity!

That Thanksgiving day in 1983 was still a year and a half before I got sober, but it was the day I went vegetarian. The gentle philosophies of recovery from addiction, like *easy does it, this too shall pass, breathe, one day at a time,* are the guiding principles of the Vegan 1 Day project.

There are many valid and important reasons to go plant-based, such as for better health, a more sustainable environment, and compassion for animals, but I believe that adopting a *one-day at a time* attitude will help prevent feeling powerless and immobile by what seems like an overwhelming transition. The mind always amplifies difficulties as being bigger than they actually are.

I am also reminded that the mind wants to give up way before the body as I continue paddling the west shore of Lake Tahoe. Locals refer to the west shore of Lake Tahoe as the "best shore." Small town feel, more open space. But for me, the west shore is the no-rest-shore. It is the beginning of the most difficult part of the paddle around the lake. As I approach Sugar Pine Point, my feet, which have been partially numb for the last two hours, start to cramp with spasms. It's my arches. Also, I encounter another head wind of about 4 mph. I move my toes and feet up and down as I paddle into the wind, first lifting my toes, then my heel as high as I can, one foot at a time. The side chop from wind and speedboats, my fatigue, and the narrow aspect of my SUP board make for a difficult moment to release tension from my legs and feet. The stretching helps, but the wind doesn't let up.

Every single negative thought I could imagine thinking of occurs every year along the west shore of Lake Tahoe on these paddle expeditions.

I think, for example that... my feet will stop working, my arms will stop working, headwind will build and will become too strong for me to continue, I will suddenly forget how to balance, rain and thunderstorms will come, I will become too nauseous to continue, the Vegan 1 Day message is too naive, too idealistic, nobody cares, I am weak, I will fall asleep and lose my board, there is no hope. Well, you get the idea.

As soon as I recognize that I'm thinking a negative thought, I replace it with a positive one. I replace... my arms will stop working, with my arms are working right now. I replace.... I am weak with have fun. The thunderstorms will kill me with look at the beautiful clouds.

The instant liberation of transforming the negative into positive is completely energizing. It's astonishing how much stronger I feel after losing hope, letting go of expectation, not caring about outcome! For me, the paddle around the lake is a journey within. Being alone in the unresolved wilderness of myself, I cease fighting and find peace. My past addictions have only been distractions from myself. They were fun, pitiful, mind-blowing, horrible, sad, happy, tragic, journeys away from my heart. That's what I did, until I stopped doing it.

Paddling alone, the fatigue bounces around in my mind and body like an echo chamber. There is no one there to help diffuse the powerful incoming messages of *I can't*, and *it's too difficult*. For me, the overcoming of difficulty always helps me have more compassion for others.

I've heard people tell me that they would die, not figuratively speaking, literally die, if they didn't eat meat. People say that they could never give up eating cheese. What about family traditions? I've heard, "I can't help it, I just love the taste of meat," or, "When I go to a baseball game in L.A., I hear Vin Scully's voice and I want a Dodger dog," or, "The smell of bacon makes me happy." I get it! I've been there. In my early months of sobriety, I would binge on bags of nacho cheese Doritos with melted cheddar cheese on top. Not drinking, no problem! I'm not even thinking about it, as I take the tray of two bags of cheese-drenched Doritos out of the oven.

Food has a powerful emotional component. Perhaps food can be as strong as a drug is for an addict. Our society is hooked on meat, dairy and eggs, but we don't want to admit it.

Dr. Neal Barnard writes in the book, *Breaking the Food Seduction*, about the habit-forming nature of animal foods and in particular, how dairy has a narcotic effect on the brain. We're a pack-a-day smoker saying that we can quit at any time, but we tell ourselves that we just don't want to today.

Or, perhaps it's as simple as people doing what others around them are doing. As is said, the reason why people eat meat is because the people around them eat meat. And so the beat goes on.

With cramped feet, and a headwind, I hit the proverbial wall at Homewood, just past Sugar Pine Point. I give up caring about if I will make it all the way around the lake. I see families on the shore in Homewood enjoying the beautiful day, and I notice it IS indeed a beautiful day to be on the lake! Enjoy the paddle, and keep going! The mind wants to give up way before the body. When hitting a wall, there is always a rebound. They call it riding the pink cloud. This particularly wonderful pink cloud wrapped its arms around me and carried me for ten miles.

Ten miles is plenty of time to focus my mind on a spiritual mantra. When I'm feeling good, or when I'm feeling bad, or none of the above, I chant the Maha-Mantra. Seventy-two miles around Lake Tahoe, and all that the expedition brings up, is the perfect opportunity for mantra meditation. I prefer prayer, meditation, and the natural sounds of the lake to wearing headphones with music.

The good vibrations lasted all the way past Tahoe City, around Dollar point, past Carnelian Bay, and into Kings Beach. Then, Bam! I hit another wall. Hello sweetheart. In the blink of an eye, the beauty of my surroundings look drab and worn out. Gone is the clarity in my vision. The sky has lost its splendor to me, and the lake now feels like cement. I reach down to filter more drinking water from the lake. I know that the low feeling will pass again, so I let it. Just as quickly as exhaustion and despair arrive, they vanish, after which I feel as chipper as a hummingbird in a flower. Now, I'm only miles from home. I feel good! I feel really good! Emerald-Bay-around-the-island-twice-kind-of-good!

The undulating waves of strength-exhaustion-exhaustion-strength, and the accompanying hope-despair yo-yo during endurance paddles are a trip. My shoulders and hips are tight and sore, but I have renewed energy, and a metaphorical new pair of glasses. A vibrant green color of the Jeffery pine trees now framing the lake brilliantly offsets the blueness of the mountain sky. I pass Speedboat Beach with strokes as powerful as ever. I feel as strong as Popeye on a two-day spinach bender.

The lake is full of boaters, other stand up paddlers, kayakers, and people enjoying the beaches. It's a warm, summer day. A woman on a SUP sees my long board, shoulder hydration pack, and determined look and says, "Oh, you look serious, where you going'?" "Incline Village," I say, giving a nodding motion with my head.

I purposefully exclude the details of taking the LONG way around to Incline Village, paddling at night, demons in Homewood, two laps around Emerald Bay island, Seventy two miles non-stop, "do the best you can," cramps, depression, elation, "go Vegan 1 Day," parts of the story while answering her question. She says, "Oh, that's not too far, have fun!" Smiling, I say, "Thanks, enjoy the day." I put my head down and paddle, picking up the pace. I have four miles to go. I can taste it.

The last four miles are a piece of cake, a piece of raw-vegan, sugar-free, date, pecan, cashew cream cake (one of which I hope to enjoy very soon!). Delightful! The beach at Incline Village, my destination, grows larger and larger in my vision. My strength also grows larger and larger until.... home, sweet home!

I hop off my board into the shallow water at Ski Beach in Incline Village. I dig my feet into the sand as feeling starts to return to my toes. I dive underwater. Bathing in the beauty of the crystal clear waters of Lake Tahoe and the blissful buzz of stillness now pumping through my veins. It's been a long day, a full day. The successive moments strung together in a circle that is the beauty of Lake Tahoe, bringing me here again into this moment. The angelic sight of Carol, on the beach, appears to me, like an apparition of the Virgin of Guadalupe. Beautiful.

I look at my watch. 5:45 p.m. It takes a moment for me to gather my thoughts, trying to figure out how long the paddle actually took to complete. The mental logjam of my fatigued mind amuses me. I end up using my fingers to count the hours from when I started at 3:30 a.m. Fourteen hours and fifteen minutes total. I can't believe it! That's my fastest time so far, a half an hour faster than the previous year. In fact, fourteen hours and fifteen minutes is exactly the same time as a World Record accomplishment by an outrigger canoe paddler named Grant Korgan, who set out to break the world record for fastest human powered non-stop circumnavigation of Lake Tahoe. Grant had a companion SUP paddler, a friend of mine named Adam Freeman, who confirmed his accomplishment. I had no one to confirm either my route or time so Grant's record book accomplishment still stands alone.

The joy of living life to the fullest is my motivation for paddling the entirety of the lake, but I can't lie, I am also a competitive person. In an instant, with the thought of the speed of my paddle and the comparison with others, I'm transported away from the miracle of living into struggle and competition.

I've been athletic and have surfed my entire life. In my thirties, when I started surfing bigger and bigger waves in Northern California and Southern Baja, naturally the famous big wave location of Mavericks, in Half Moon Bay, California, captured my imagination, and needed to be surfed. And now, in my fifties, I still race in competitive SUP races. I suppose I relate to the mythical Don Quixote tilting at windmills.

It's good for me to note the time it took to complete the circumnavigation, recognizing a meaningless unofficial record of sorts, and it is also good for me to let it go, giving it wings! I am a good example of how our world is focused on results. We are fascinated with the end of the story, but less by the method or the course of the journey. I am reminded again and again, year after year; as I paddle the entirety of Lake Tahoe to seek the joy in the process, experience the wonderment of each and every moment, not the waiting for what comes next.

Ultimately, this is the message of the Vegan 1 Day project. Enjoy the journey! Live one day at a time, taking each day as it comes. Try going vegan one day a week, one day a month, or all the time, your choice! Learn about new, healthier plant-based foods. Learn about how animals are treated in the meat industry and about the environmental effects of animal agriculture. If these practices don't align with your values, why support them?

The Hindu scripture, Bhagavad-Gita reminds us that meaningful change comes from the inside out, not the outside in. Perhaps our inability to sustain our aspirations is due to our outward perspective, usually filled with our expectations, judgments of right and wrong, good and bad, doubts, fears, and frustrations.

When there is so much at stake—better health, more environmental sustainability, and less animal suffering, why do we imagine that adopting a plant-based diet is so difficult?

When we shift our awareness to our inner experience, we can navigate with meaning and purpose. Inwardly, we can reflect on our own obstructions and how to overcome them. Compassion for animals is the same source of compassion we must have for ourselves. Taking it day by day, we're all capable of change. There is power, and freedom, living in the moment. It's not about how fast or slow we go around Big Blue; it's about that we don't stop paddling.

The question for you then becomes, is Vegan 1 Day today?

Setting Up a Compassionate Kitchen

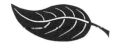

*"If one offers me with love and devotion, a leaf, a flower,
fruit, or water, I will accept it."*

~ Krsna

The Magic Magnifying Mind

Energy flows where our attention goes. We have magic-magnifying minds. If we focus on the positive, the positive will grow. If we focus on the negative, the negative will grow. By choosing whole, plant-based foods, you are likely to enjoy delicious food, improve your health, help the environment, and cause less suffering to animals. Sounds pretty good, right? But if you focus on how difficult change is or on all of the foods you cannot eat.... Bingo! Your experience can be predicted.

The best place to start is right where you are. Take a look around your kitchen. You probably eat many plant-based foods already. Fruits, vegetables, grains, beans, nuts – all of these foods are vegan.

Veganizing a kitchen is simple. Opening our minds to the simplicity is one of the best parts of the adventure of creating a healthier life and a healthier world.

You may have questions about what's it's like to eat a vegan diet. Is it difficult? What about when eating out at restaurants? Can I go vegan, except for having non-vegan cake at a party? Will my friends and family accept my choice to eat vegan? All of these and other questions have to do with your own journey to find what's true for you in each moment that arises. There are no rules to follow. You don't have to know everything to start. Making a beginning will open the door for a clearer view of a more compassionate path.

When choosing healthy plant-based foods we cause less harm and that goodness returns to us in ways that are seen and in ways that are unseen, as well. We are what we eat. Living a good life starts with a mindful connection with the world around us and with the food we eat.

It will be helpful to learn about plant-based foods; where they come from, what they are, how to get them, and how to prepare them. It will also be helpful to read the labels of ingredients on packaged foods in order to be truly informed as to what you are putting into your body.

If this sounds like a lot, then take baby steps. Even the smallest steps to go vegan are big steps. Think of it as an adventure. But remember, nothing changes if nothing changes.

When challenges arise, bring to mind the benefits of having a compassionate kitchen. Whole plant-based foods are healthier than animal foods, more sustainable for our environment, and cause less harm to animals.

The recipes we provide are plant-based alternatives to meat, dairy and eggs. These recipes are offered here to inspire and sustain a vegan path, but remember, keep it simple. When you're ready, take a look at some of the recipes in this book to help replace the non-vegan dishes with plant-based alternatives. You'll be amazed by the flavors and fullness you experience from a vegan way of life.

The Humane Myth

A lot of well-intentioned people who want to set up a compassionate kitchen are under the impression that it's fine to consume meat, dairy, and eggs as long as it is raised humanely. The question that comes to mind is what are the standards that qualify as humane?

Can the reality of a slaughterhouse and the ethos of humane treatment of animals be considered congruent? All so-called humanely raised grass-fed cattle, free-range chickens, and dairy cows ultimately end up at slaughterhouses.

Also, some people may not be aware of the crowding that is still allowable under humane certification. Some animals cannot even go outside, and common mutilations such as cutting off the beaks of chickens are allowed in "humane" industry. The "humane" egg industry and back-yard chicken enthusiasts unwittingly support egg hatcheries where babies never see their mothers and males are destroyed and thrown into the trash at birth. They also might not know that hens don't lay eggs their entire lives. So when their egg production declines or stops, they too are slaughtered.

Once, a friend of ours in Baja jokingly referred to us as a couple of "do-gooders." At the time it was sort of a back-handed compliment, but it is a fair characterization.

When did "doing good" become a bad thing? In a

culture where the commodification of animals is so deeply entrenched in our unconscious that the notion of humane treatment includes killing animals so we can eat them, we realize that there is a long way to go. We can use a lot more do-gooders in the world! For us, a plant-based diet is an opportunity to practice kindness and compassion. When examining whether something is humane, we would ask the question, would we want it done to us?

Where Do You Get Protein?

One of the most common misperceptions about a plant-based diet is that it is somehow lacking sufficient protein. Protein is the keystone of human nutrition and is not to be overlooked, but it is virtually impossible to *not* get enough protein from a plant-based diet if your caloric intake is sufficient. In other words, if you eat enough food, you will get enough protein.

According to the Journal of Academy of Nutrition and Dietetics, *Study of the nutrient profiles of vegetarians and non-vegetarians dietary patterns,* virtually everyone (whether plant-based or omnivore) gets 30% more than adequate levels of protein, based on the FDA's recommended daily intake.

So, it makes us wonder, why all of the focus on protein? We are, quite literally, protein-obsessed.

Americans are highly concerned about protein intake, yet they are among some of the least healthy in the world. According to World Health Organization studies, the United States ranks higher in rates of obesity, diabetes, heart disease, and some forms of cancer than many less developed countries.

Dr. Garth Davis, author of the book *Proteinaholic*, postulates that our protein obsession has caused an overall less healthy population. "After years of intense research, I could come to only one conclusion: People whose diets are high in *animal* protein have significantly higher rates of chronic diseases: hypertension, cancer, diabetes, heart disease, and many, many others, including cataracts, diverticulitis, diverticulosis, inflammatory bowel disease, gall bladder disorders, gout, hypertension, irritable bowel syndrome, kidney stones and rheumatoid arthritis. That's what I know for certain."

Since most people view animal foods as their primary source for protein, the American obsession with protein can be translated into, *"eat meat kids, it's good for you."* Meanwhile, those kids are growing into sick, unhealthy adults with one foot in the grave. One of Dr. Davis' conclusions is that protein is not only commonly available in plant-based food, it is much better for us than animal protein.

Much of what people have learned about protein has been sold to them by the meat industry. "Milk, it does a body good" or "Beef, it's what's for dinner" ad campaigns include information about the amount of protein per serving of milk or beef, and has subconsciously embedded itself into our psyche. The public, as well as some of the established medical community, have bought this myth hook, line, and sinker. The lack of knowledge about the abundance of protein in a plant-based diet is extraordinary.

Here is the protein content of some plant-based foods:

Name	Amount	Protein (G)
Almonds	1/4 C	8.0
Apple	1 C	1.0
Apricot	1 C	2.31
Artichoke	1 C	3.47
Arugula	1 C	5.16
Asparagus	1/4 C	4.32
Avocado	1 C	4.02
Banana	1 C	1.64
Beet	1 C	2.19
Black Beans	1 C	15.24
Blackberries	1 C	2.0
Blueberries	1 C	1.1
Broccoli	1 C	2.57
Brown Rice	1 C	4.52
Brussels Sprouts	1 C	4.0
Buckwheat	1 C	5.68
Butternut Squash	1 C	1.84
Cabbage	1 C	1.14
Cantaloupe	1 C	1.49
Carrots	1 C	1.19
Cashews	1 C	11.0
Cauliflower	1 C	2.05
Chia Seeds	1 oz.	4.69
Chickpeas	1 C	14.53
Cocoa Powder	1 C	17.0
Cucumber	1 C	1.0
Eggplant	1 C	.83
Figs	1 C	1.5
Flax Seed	1 C	7.6

Grapefruit	1 C	1.45
Green Beans	1C	1.83
Green Peas	1 C	1.83
Hemp Seed	3 TBS	9.0
Kale	1 C	2.21
Kidney Beans	1 C	7.73
Kiwi	1 C	2.05
Lentils	1 C	18.0
Macadamia Nuts	1 C	10.6
Maca Root Powder	1 TBS	4.0
Mango	1 C	1.06
Medjool Dates	1 C	1.72
Millet	1 C	6.11
Miso	1 TBS	2.0
Mixed Greens	1 C	.5
Mustard Greens	1 C	2.0
Nut Butter (Almonds)	1 C	16.0
Nut Butter (Cashew)	1 C	12.0
Nutritional Yeast	1/4 C	16.0
Oatmeal	1 C	14.0
Orange	1 C	1.23
Parsley	1 C	1.8
Peach	1 C	1.36
Pecans	1/4 C	5.0
Pine Nuts	1/2 C	9.24
Pumpkin Seeds	1/2 C	19.5
Raspberries	1 C	1.48
Red Pepper	1 C	1.18
Quinoa	1 C	24.0
Sesame Seeds	1 C	6.38
Spinach	1 C	.86

Spirulina	1 TBS.	4.0
Strawberries	1 C	.96
Sunflower Seeds	1 C	9.56
Sweet Potato	1 C	2.29
Tahini	1/4 C	12.0
Tomatoes	1 C	1.08
Walnuts	1 C	8.0
Watercress	1 C	1.0
Watermelon	1 C	1.74
Wild Rice	1 C	7.0
Yellow Squash	1 C	1.28
Zucchini	1 C	1.87

(Source: USDA, National Nutrient Database)

For many people, transitioning to a plant-based diet can kick up the dust of addictions. Addiction is when our cravings drive us to do something that we know is not good for us but we do it anyway.

Sometimes people who are new to a vegan diet can confuse a craving for animal foods with the notion that animal protein is needed to be healthy. In actuality, their habituation to animal protein has all of the hallmarks of addiction.

Dr. Neal Barnard, noted physician and author of the book, *Breaking the Food Seduction* says, "The most important thing to understand about cravings: They are not caused by weak will or gluttony. Cravings are triggered by biological properties of the foods themselves. That is, certain foods have chemical makeups that cause us to crave them in very much the same way that drugs, alcohol, and tobacco have addictive components."

Most people may not identify themselves as being addicted to animal foods. They see themselves as simply enjoying the taste of their favorite meal, accommodating the desires of their appetite, or trying to meet their nutritional needs. Yet, with a growing scientific consensus about the health benefits of a plant-based diet and a growing understanding about the negative impacts of animal agriculture and the destructiveness to our planet, you would assume people would switch to a plant-based diet straight away!

The truth is animal foods are addictive and change is not easy, but there is hope. People are waking up to the false narratives of the meat industry. They are slowly learning about plant-based foods, which are becoming more and more convenient to purchase.

One of the most significant things we'd like you to keep in mind is as we change, so does our taste. Dr. Barnard goes on to say, "The taste buds have a memory of about three weeks." Our actual taste for food changes as we evolve and eat healthier foods, and as our taste changes, so does our experience. One of our spiritual teachers, Srila Prahbupada, describes the process of developing a new sense experience with food as a *higher taste*.

To us, nothing tastes better than health-promoting, plant-based (protein abundant) foods prepared with love. But the vegan path might take time. Don't beat yourself up if you crave meat or cheese at the very moment you decide to go vegan. It happens. You're not alone, nor are you the first person to have extracted yourself from the grasp of the meat industry. The important thing to remember is that a path with purpose always has obstacles to overcome.

A friend of mine named Steve, who calls himself an

omnivore, said to me, "I could never go vegan because I couldn't give up cheese." I suggested to him that he should go vegan, except for cheese. Just for the record, he hasn't yet tried any of the incredible plant-based cheeses like Daiya or Miyoko, and if he does, he may think otherwise.

But the point is, there is nothing wrong with going *vegan-ish*. The more you open the door to healthier foods, the healthier you will become, and then, the more you will want to open the door for more healthy foods.

Think of it as a spiral staircase going up. You start to see the view the higher you go.

Organico!

Organic foods are delicious and are also packed with more nutrition than conventionally grown foods. They are GMO free and most importantly, organic farming excludes pesticides and herbicides which cause harm to the environment (as well as our health). Farmers' markets will have the fruits and vegetables that are in season in your region, or start growing your own food! Carol and I have mango, avocado, lemon, papaya, and grapefruit trees on our property in Baja. We also grow spinach, arugula and kale in our local community garden, all organic.

Stuff

Here is a list of kitchen appliances that some of our recipes call for.

- *Blender* (We love our Vitamix and use it every day, but other blender brands are also fine.)

- *Juicer* (Masticating is best, but anything will work. We use it several times a week.)

- *Food processor* (We use it every so often)

Good Foods

Here are some foods we love (and use often) when preparing recipes:

Avocado - tastes great, and is nutrient-dense with healthy fats. Avocado are very versatile, and can be used with many foods, including desserts and smoothies. We eat at least one avocado a day.

Beans (black, pinto, lentil, mung, adzuki) - These are highly nutritious, no cholesterol and versatile to cook with, and are also low on the glycemic scale, so they don't cause blood-sugar spikes. These are a staple in our diet.

Greens - Kale, arugula, parsley, cilantro, spinach, mint, Swiss chard, romaine, bok choy, basil, sprouts. These are good in smoothies, juices, salads, soups, and are packed full of nutrition. Greens are another staple of our diet.

Yams and Sweet Potatoes - They are a good (and inexpensive) source of nutrition, high in protein, and fiber.

Whole Grains - (oats, quinoa, brown rice, barley, millet, buckwheat, corn) We use these hardy foods, mixing them with veggies, beans, and greens.

Chia seeds - They're a great source of healthy omega-3 fatty acids, high in anti-oxidants, and are a significant source of bio-available protein. We use these in pudding and with oatmeal.

Hemp seeds - Similar to chia seeds; these are high in omega-3 fatty acids and protein. These are good in smoothies and as a topper on salads.

Spirulina - One of the most nutrient-dense foods on the planet. It is a fresh-water blue green algae, highly digestible and bio-available. It is a complete protein with all the essential amino acids, as well as being high in omega-3 fatty acids. It's a terrific aid for endurance events. It's good in smoothies and as a juice drink.

Wheatgrass Juice - This is a highly nutritious power-packed throw-it-back-in-a-shot-glass juice, which can help stimulate and regulate blood and thyroid function.

Maca - A root native to the high Andes of Peru. It's an endurance booster, increasing oxygen intake and sustaining energy. John first discovered maca while traveling in Peru where Peruvian porters would drink maca tea and chew coca leaves while on (relatively) high altitude expeditions with him. It's good in smoothies and as a tea.

Tofu and Tempeh (tempeh is fermented soy) - These are very versatile foods for cooking, and are highly bio-available sources of protein, calcium, minerals, and vitamins, including vitamin K.

Fermented Foods - Along with the above mentioned tempeh, there are other fermented live foods, like kombucha, sauerkraut, kimchi, and miso that promote a healthy gut ecology by providing probiotic digestive enzymes, increased nutrients, and enhanced immunity. These fermented foods assist us with healthy digestion and maximum absorption of all the wonderful nutrient-dense greens, fruits, veggies and herbs we eat.

Fruit - You name it, we eat it. Papaya, pineapple, pears, mango, jackfruit, apple, kiwi, banana, coconut, strawberries, blueberries, blackberries, goji berries, mulberries, raspberries, grapes, figs, dates, orange, lime, lemon, grapefruit, tomatoes... Fresh organic fruits are a staple of our diet.

Vegetables - Cauliflower, broccoli, carrots, beets, bell peppers, cucumbers, celery... We use these in soups, smoothies, stir-fries, steamed, and more.

Turmeric - This is a yellow spice common in Indian foods. It is a powerful antioxidant and anti-inflammatory. It aids in pain relief and recovery while training. It is also thought to protect our cells from certain forms of cancer. It's good in curries, tea, and soups.

Supplements - The only supplement we take is a (sublingual) B-12 spray, once a day. B-12 is the only vitamin in short supply in a plant-based diet. All other vitamins and nutrients (including iron and calcium) we obtain in more than adequate quantities from a whole food, plant-based diet.

Food at the Market

Here is a list of store bought plant-based foods to help replace meat, dairy and eggs. Many of these plant-based companies understand the value of organic as well as delivering a product with as minimal processing as possible so we can recommend these plant-based alternatives. They are convenient and easy to serve and more than just replicating the taste of meat, dairy and eggs. In many cases they taste superior and are healthier, as well as compassionate to animals.

- Hot Dogs: Field Roast, Tofurky (organic), Yves
- Hamburgers: Amy's Kitchen (organic), Beyond Meat, Gardein, Sunshine
- Pork: Gardein
- Seafood: Sophie's Kitchen
- Sausage: Amy's Kitchen, Tofurky (organic), Field Roast
- Beef: Beyond Meat, Gardein, Tofurky (organic), Field Roast
- Cheese: Daiya, Miyoko Creamery, Nacheez, Vegan Gourmet
- Eggs: Ener-G, Follow Your Heart, Vegg

- Milk: (soy, hemp, almond, rice, cashew, etc.) So Delicious, Silk, West Soy (organic)
- Yogurt: So Delicious (Coconut vanilla unsweetened)
- Mayonnaise: Hampton Creek-just mayo, Follow Your Heart- veganaise
- Butter: Earth Balance

If your local market doesn't carry these products, ask the manager to stock them, or you can special order them as well.

Living the Good Life

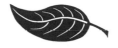

"Easy does it."

~ Anonymous

For us, living vegan is a celebration of life. It's a joy to learn about and search for healthy, cruelty-free foods. Eating consciously is one of the greatest gifts we've given ourselves and the world around us.

However, going vegan is not without its challenges. Changing our eating habits in a world where the status quo is reinforced and even rewarded through marketing and social norms, there are bound to be challenges. Whatever challenges you may encounter while going vegan (or even vegan-ish), if they are met with an adventurous spirit and a compassionate heart, they can easily be overcome. Know that you're not alone. We are with you and we are for you every step of the way!

Thank you for caring enough to read this book. The animals thank you for caring about making changes to your food choices.

We support you on your own path to living the good life. We hope you find the abundance of a vegan way of life and the beauty of living one day at a time.

~ Carol and John

Vegan 1 Day Recipes

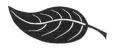

The recipes in this book are some of our favorites. They are healthy and delicious. We have a Vegan 1 Day community of friends who have also contributed some of their recipes as well. We hope you enjoy them.

~ Carol and John

Alida Labia's Recipe for Going Vegan

First, visit Animal Place or Farm Sanctuary, where animals are seen as individuals. Observe and meditate with chickens and turkeys as they dust bathe, croon melodies, and observe you curiously looking back. Become infatuated with a rooster named Errol, who loves sitting on your lap. He is partial to many laps, so you could be next to fall under his spell. Look into the soft intelligent eyes of Wilbur the pig, and feed him fruit salad. Get chased by goats Noah and Cornelius, and a donkey named Jellybean, quite exhilarating! Marvel at the gentleness of the sheep whilst sitting on a rock listening to them grazing. Laugh at the playfulness of rescued calves, Shelby and Magnolia. Feel gratitude sitting with the bunnies, some of whom have been saved from the horrible life in a laboratory. Mix all these pleasures together, and enjoy!

Having the privilege of spending time with farmed animals, animals whom are thought of by most people as food, is a joy. They are just like us, wanting to enjoy their lives, to express themselves, nurture their young and be with friends and sniff the air. Simply put, go vegan, for the animals, and yourself.

Malinalco Turmeric Tea

½ cup water
¼ turmeric (ground)
¼ black pepper (ground)
1 teaspoon coconut oil

Heat in a small saucepan until it becomes a watery paste. You want it to be a little watery, because when it's saved in the refrigerator, the paste thickens.

For two cups of tea-
2 teaspoons of the turmeric paste (that you made in the saucepan)
2 large cups of plant-based milk (almond, soy, rice, etc.)
4 dates (pitted)

Blend well in a Vitamix blender.
Heat, and enjoy!

Paddle-All-Day-Green-Juice

Kale
Celery
Mango
Watermelon
Maca
Spirulina

Amounts vary to your taste.

Run the kale, celery, and mango through the Juicer, and add the maca and spirulina powder to the mix.

Put it in your shoulder hydration pack, and now go paddle!

Green Smoothies

SEA OF CORTEZ
Cilantro (large hand full)
1 avocado
Watermelon
1 Orange
2 cups of water

TAHOE BLUE BERRIES
Spinach (large hand full)
½ cup of Blueberries
2 Bananas
2 cups of water

REALLY ARUGULA
Arugula (large hand full)
2 Apples
2 bananas
Ginger (small slice)
2 cups of water

WILD MINT
Mint (1 bunch)
Kale (2 large leaves)
Pear (4)
2 cups of water

Chia-Seed-Surf-All-Morning-Pudding

½ cup chia seed
1 tsp. cinnamon
5 pitted Medjool dates
Almond Milk

Vitamix almond milk and pitted dates- leave chunky (put as much almond milk in to your taste. Let stand for 15 minutes so chia seeds soak up the almond milk)

Add:
2 chopped figs
some chopped almonds
shredded coconut
mulberries
a little coconut oil
cacao nibs
Enjoy!
Now go surf!

Carol's No Name Oatmeal

Boil whole oats
Add:
almond (or peanut butter),
raisins,
cinnamon,
apple (or any fruit),
walnuts
Soy or almond milk
Enjoy!
Now go to Saturday garage sales!

Hummus

1 can of garbanzo beans
4 tbs. tahini
¼ cup of water
2 tbs. lemon juice
½ tsp. cumin
½ tsp. salt
Blend well
Enjoy!

Guacamole

4 avocados (ripe)
1 tsp. Spike seasoning
½ onion (chopped)
Some squeezed lemon or lime
½ bunch of cilantro (chopped)
½ small Serrano pepper (finely chopped)
1 large tomato (chopped)
Smash the avocado, and mix the other ingredients together with the avocado. Enjoy!

Loretta's Cowboy Caviar (Loretta Hitch)

(2) 1 oz. cans of white corn (drained)
(2) 15 oz. cans of black-eyed peas (drained)
1 bunch of cilantro (chopped)
1 bunch of green onion (chopped)
1/3 cup of olive oil
2-3 avocados (diced)
2-3 Roma tomatoes (chopped)
2-3 garlic cloves (crushed)
1 tsp. ground cumin
½ cup red wine vinegar
Mix all ingredients together well, add Valentina salsa to taste, enjoy!

Pea Spread on Toast

1 bag frozen peas
2 crushed garlic cloves
2 tbsp. olive oil
Salt and Pepper (4 turns on the grinder each)
Vegan cheese (Daiya) ¼ to ½ cup
Bread for toast (2-4 slices)
Fresh mint (chopped)

1. Boil a pot of water; when at full boil add frozen peas, cover and take off of heat.
2. Let sit in hot water 5 minutes. Drain and let cool.
3. Mash peas and then add the garlic, olive oil, and cheese. Salt and pepper to taste.
4. Toast bread and cut into 4 quarters.
5. Spread pea mixture on toast and sprinkle mint on top.

Enjoy!

Jicama Salad Tacos

1 small jicama (cut into strips)
½ red pepper (cut into strips)
1 small yellow chile (diced)
1 orange
½ cup rice vinegar
1 cup walnuts (chopped fine)
½ pomegranate (seeds only)
red cabbage leaves

Add all ingredients together in a bowl, except the orange. Cut orange in half. Squeeze ½ of the orange into the bowl with other ingredients. Chop the other half of the orange into small squares and add to the bowl. Mix and put ingredients in red cabbage leaves (like a taco). Enjoy!

Yolanda's Rainbow Summer Salad (Yolanda Labia)

2 cups chopped green cabbage
1 cup chopped red cabbage
1 bok choy chopped
3 stalks of celery chopped
3 grated carrots
1/2 red pepper chopped
2 tablespoons of raw pumpkin seeds
2 table spoons of raw sunflower seeds
1 tablespoon of sesame seeds
1 cup of steamed or sprouted lentils
1/2 cup of dried currants.
Salad Dressing
Your choice - but I use a balsamic vinaigrette to keep it "light"
like summer.

There is currently a mania in the food-marketing arena regarding animal based protein. It is important to realize that less than 1% of the population is protein deficient in comparison to the 97% that is fiber deficient. Fiber can only be sourced in plant foods and is essential for digestive health, cardiovascular health and blood sugar control.

So go ahead and enjoy my Summer Salad. It's packed with fiber!

Collard Rice Wraps (Monica Quinones)

These wraps make a wonderful lunch or dinner and are good hot or cold. This recipe could make about 6 wraps, but that really depends on leaf size as they can range from small to huge! Collard green leaves make wonderful wraps; they're mild in flavor yet strong enough to not wilt when wrapped in foil for a packed meal on the go.

Ingredients:
collard green leaves
1 cup uncooked grain (brown rice or barley)
1/2 cup uncooked quinoa
juice & zest from 2 lemons
1 cucumber, thinly sliced
1 tsp dried oregano
tahini
hot sauce of choice (I like Crystal for these)

Method:
Add grain and quinoa to medium pot with 2 cups water. Bring to a boil, then reduce heat to low and cover. Allow cooking 20-30 minutes. Meanwhile wash your collard green leaves and carefully thin center stem with sharp knife, then set aside. In large mixing bowl, combine thinly sliced cucumber, lemon juice, lemon zest and oregano. When the grain/quinoa mix has fully cooked, add to other ingredients in mixing bowl and stir well. Spread a generous amount of tahini onto collard green leaf and top with rice mixture. Lastly add hot sauce of choice. Wrap it up and enjoy!

Green Goddess Griller (Keaven Van Lom)

Note: Probably "the best" sandwich I have ever had!

Pesto:
> 1/3 cup basil
> 1/4 cup pine nuts
> 1-2 garlic cloves
> 1 cup kale, chopped, deveined
> 1/4 cup (or more) of olive oil
> Salt and pepper to taste

Sandwich:
> Sourdough bread (my favorite, or Spelt, wheat, etc.)
> 1/2 avocado, sliced
> 1/2 cup spinach
> Your favorite vegan cheese (I like creamy Chao)
> Vegan or coconut butter

Preparation:
1. To make the pesto, add all ingredients to blender and combine till smooth.
2. Spread pesto on both sides of bread and butter on one side, place in pan.
3. On the buttered slice add cheese, avocado, and spinach.
4. Top with other slice, press together and add butter to other slice.
5. Grill on both sides.

Karma-free Cauliflower, Pea Pods, and Cashews

3 cups cauliflower (cut into flowerets)
2 cups Chinese pea pods (remove ends)
½ cup whole cashews
1 cup vegan sour cream
1 tsp. salt
½ tsp. black pepper
pinch of turmeric
pinch of hing

In a wok, fry cauliflower pieces over medium-high heat in olive oil until golden and tender. Add cashews and pea pods for the last minute in the wok. Combine pea pods, cauliflower, cashews, and sour cream. Add spices. Heat in saucepan for 1 minute. Serve hot. Serves 2. Enjoy!

Tahoe Lentil Loaf

Cook 1½ cups of rinsed lentils in 3½ cups of water until tender. Partially mash lentils and mix with 2 medium onions that have been sautéed in a little water.

Add to the onions and lentils:
2 cups cooked rice
1 tsp. garlic powder
1 tsp. salt
¼ cup of vegan catsup
1 tsp. sage
½ tsp. marjoram

Press into a sprayed loaf pan and spread catsup over the top. Bake for 1 hour at 350 degrees. Serve and enjoy!

V Tempeh Rueben (Vee Lewin)

Ingredients:
One 8 oz. package Tempeh, sliced into sandwich sized pieces
½ cup water
1/3 cup tamari
1 teaspoon cumin
½ teaspoon caraway
2 teaspoons grainy mustard
1 clove garlic, minced
1 cup Sauerkraut, well drained,
1 cup Daiya cheese shreds
3 Tablespoons vegan mayonnaise
3 Tablespoons ketchup
3 Tablespoons pickle relish
1 large tomato, sliced thin
1 medium red onion
Sandwich bread, sliced thin, toasted

Method of Preparation:
Preheat oven to 350 degrees. In small bowl combine water, tamari, cumin, caraway, mustard, and garlic; whisk together. Place tempeh in a baking dish and place marinade over it. Bake in oven uncovered for 40 minutes. When finished cooking tempeh will be dark and should be removed from any excess liquid. Place on a separate dish and set aside. Spread drained Sauerkraut in a small frying pan and top with cheese shreds. Cover and heat over LOW heat to warm through until cheese melts.

In a small dish make the Russian dressing by combining the vegan mayo, ketchup, and pickle relish and mixing thoroughly.

Now to assemble this tasty sandwich: Place bread on a plate. Spread a tablespoon of the Russian dressing on and add the tempeh. Add the warmed Sauerkraut and cheese, then tomato, and onion and place the other piece of bread on top. Serves 4. Enjoy!

Pea and Carrot Coconut Curry

In a large frying pan, sauté 1 small onion, chopped; 1 to 2 tbsp. Madras curry powder; 1 tsp. salt; 1 chopped Serrano chile in a little vegetable oil. Add 1 lb. baby carrots, cut lengthwise; 1 cup frozen peas; ½ cup of water; and 1 can (14.5 oz.) coconut milk. Simmer, covered, until carrots are tender. Serve over steamed basmati rice and sprinkle with chopped cilantro. Enjoy!

Roasted Cauliflower with Capers

1 TBSP olive oil
2 heads cauliflower (2 lbs. each), halved and sliced thinly
½ salt
1 TBSP drained and rinsed capers, chopped
1 TBSP chopped flat-leaf parsley

1. Preheat oven to 400 degrees. Brush a rimmed baking sheet with oil. Spread cauliflower on pan. Bake until browned and edges are starting to crisp, turning once halfway through, about 45 minutes. Sprinkle with salt.
2. Transfer cauliflower to a large serving dish. Sprinkle with capers and parsley. Serve and enjoy!

Baked Ziti

12 ounces penne pasta
4 TBSP fresh basil
1 tsp salt

Herbed Ricotta:
1 1/2 cups raw macadamia nuts (soaked in water for
  4 hours)
1/8 TBSP garlic (diced)
1/2 tsp salt
1 tsp olive oil
Tomato sauce (vegan)
1 tsp olive oil
1/2 cup onion (chopped)
1 tsp garlic (diced)
3 tsp dried Italian seasoning
1 14-ounce can roasted tomatoes (diced)
1 14-ounce can tomato sauce
1 tsp salt

Cashew Cream:
1 cup raw cashews (soaked in water for 3 hours)
1/2 tsp dried oregano
1 tsp salt
2 tsp freshly squeezed lemon juice
1/4 tsp rice vinegar
3 TBSP chopped fresh parsley

Bring a pot of salted water to a boil and cook the pasta. Drain and rinse, let cool and set aside.

To make the herbed "ricotta," combine the macadamia nuts, 1/4 cup of water, the garlic, salt and olive oil in a food processor and puree for 1 minute. Scrape down the sides and purée for another   minute, until light and fluffy. Set aside.

To make the cashew cream, purée the soaked cashews in a blender until a smooth paste forms. Add 1/3 cup of water and the remaining ingredients and purée until creamy.

Preheat the oven to 350°F. To assemble the baked ziti, toss the pasta with the tomato sauce in a large bowl, and then stir in the herbed "ricotta." Mix in the cashew cream. Spread into a 9x13" baking dish, cover with aluminum foil and bake for 30 minutes, or until the cheese starts to brown. Garnish with fresh basil as desired.

Angel Hair Pasta with Walnuts and Peas

2 cups fresh peas
1 cup of walnuts
6 cloves garlic
2 tsp. olive oil
½ cup basil
½ water
7 oz. whole-wheat angel hair pasta
¼ tsp. salt
black pepper to taste
red pepper flakes to taste

1. Pre-heat oven to 350 degrees
2. Peel garlic and drizzle with olive oil. Wrap in aluminum foil and roast in oven for 30 minutes. Let cool.
3. Combine walnuts, roasted garlic, basil and water in a food processor and process for 1 minute. (Or blend until smooth.)
4. Add pasta to a pot of boiling water and cook for about 7-8 minutes (according to directions on package). Drain the pasta.
5. Toss walnut mixture with pasta. Add peas, salt, pepper, red pepper flakes. Serve and enjoy!

Freddie's Spaghetti and Tempeh Meatballs

We use whole wheat or brown rice pasta, and organic red sauce with no sugar.

For the Tempeh Meatballs
1 TBSP flax seed
3 TBSP warm water
1 block tempeh
2 shallots, chopped
2 garlic cloves
2 TBSP vegan Worcestershire sauce
2 TBSP Nutritional yeast
2 TBPS fresh parsley, chopped
1 tsp dried oregano
1 tsp dried basil
1 tsp sea salt
¼ cup plus another ¼ cup whole wheat bread crumbs
Olive oil, for frying

For the Tempeh Meatballs
Prepare the marinara sauce. In a small bowl, combine the flaxseed and warm water. Mix and let sit for about 10 minutes. This is your binder.

Break up the tempeh and add it to a food processor. Add the shallots, garlic, Worcestershire sauce, and the nutritional yeast to the food processor. Process until everything is combined.

Add the herbs and the salt to the food processor. Add the flax mixture and ¼ cup of bread crumbs to the food processor and process until well combined.

Spread the remaining ¼ cup of bread crumbs on a plate. Using a spoon, scoop up some of the tempeh mix and roll it into a ball – about the size of a golf ball. Roll the tempeh meatball in the bread crumbs so that it's completely covered and set it aside on a plate. Continue making meatballs until you use up all the tempeh mix.

Heat the oil in a large skillet over medium-high heat. Add the tempeh meatballs to the skillet and fry them. Make sure the meatballs brown on all sides. When they are browned, transfer the meatballs to a paper towel-lined plate.

Gently add the tempeh meatballs to the simmering marinara sauce. Let them cook about 10 minutes until they are heated through. Serve with pasta or in a sandwich.

Mangia!

Todos Santos Bean Soup

Cooked beans 1-2 cups (pinto or any beans you like)
6 cups water or vegetable broth
1 large white onion (diced)
2 tbsp. dried rosemary (crushed)
1 cup Brown rice (cooked)
1 large potato (chopped)
3 carrots (chopped)
2 zucchini (chopped)
3 large stalks of celery (chopped)
1 small jar roasted red peppers (diced)
Some Valentina Salsa (to taste)
3 tbsp. olive oil

Add all ingredients to a large pot. Turn up to high heat, boil for 10 minutes, stirring frequently. Reduce heat and cook for 45 minutes.
Enjoy!

Sissy's Refried Beans

2 lbs. pinto beans
2 large white onions
2 serrano peppers

Preparation:
In a large pot of water add 2 lbs. of beans, 2 large onions in big chunks, 2 Serrano peppers. Boil on low heat for approximately 3 hours or until beans are soft.

To refry the beans, sauté one diced onion in a saucepan with olive oil until starting to caramelize. Drain beans from the pot and add to saucepan and start mashing!

Buena Vista Tortilla Bake

This is a dish we bring to friend's homes and potlucks. Everyone loves it and no one can believe it's vegan.

1 Package of Beyond Meat's "Beyond Beef – Feisty Crumble"
2 cans of organic refried pinto beans
Corn Tortillas (18 or so)
Corn (1 can)
Black Olives (1 can sliced)
Green Chiles (1 small can)
Salsa (2-3 jars, non-chunky) mild or medium
Daiya Cheddar Cheese (Shredded)

Layer a glass baking dish with three layers of (in this order):
Layer of salsa
Layer of 6 tortillas
Layer of refried beans
Layer of Beyond Beef – Feisty Crumble
Layer of some corn
Layer of some olives
Layer of some Daiya Cheese
Layer of some green chiles
-Repeat (2 more layers)
Bake at 400 degrees covered for approximately 25 minutes
Serves 6

Grilled Plantain, Black Bean Tacos

4 medium ripe plantains
1 can of black beans
Corn tortillas
1 ripe avocado
Handful of cilantro
Salsa verde or any other spicy salsa you like
1 lime

Heat corn tortillas with the black beans on the grill. Brush the sliced plantains with olive oil and grill separately until heavily brown on both sides. Cut the avocado and chop the cilantro. Add all ingredients onto the corn tortillas, and add salsa verde and lime to taste.

Marinated Tofu in towel
Press: extra firm tofu 20 min.
Slice: onto cookie sheet
marinate: Braggs + ~ It. Seasonings
20 mins ~ Ginger Tumeric
~ Falafel Crust
~ anything!
Bake: 400° 20 mins

Chocolate Cream Pie (Jennifer Bodaken)

Crust:
4 cups cashews (or any nuts)
20 medjool dates
1 tsp cinnamon

Filling:
4-6 ripe avocados
20-25 medjool dates
4 TBSP cacao powder
Coconut on top (shaved)

Process the crust ingredients (nuts first until the consistency of the nut meal, then add dates and spices) until it holds together and then press into a pie pan.

Put the filing ingredients in the food processor and alter to taste as needed. Scoop into the pie shell and put in the freezer.

Mima's Mango Surprise

6 cups frozen mango
1 handful pitted dates
1 tsp vanilla
1 can unsweetened coconut milk

Blend in a Vitamix blender. Sprinkle chocolate cacao nibs, and cacao powder on top.
Serve and enjoy!

Annette's Dark Chocolate Brownies (Annette Sylbalski)

2 oz. unsweetened chocolate
½ oz. semi-sweet chocolate
2 tsp. vanilla
1 tbs rice syrup
4 tbs water or as needed
2 eggs vegan equivalent Egg Replacer Brand
3 TBSP soy protein powder *or any*
2 TBSP unsweetened cocoa powder
¼ tsp salt
¼ tsp baking soda
Sprinkle on top raisins, chunks of unsweetened chocolate and cocoa powder.
Bake at 350 degrees for 10 minutes in a square glass pan.
Enjoy!

Date Banana Ice Cream

Medjool Pitted Dates (8)
Frozen Bananas (4) or 1 banana for each person served.
Soy or Almond Milk (1/2 cup)
Peanut butter (1 tsp.)
Cacao powder (1tsp.)
Ice cubes (4 large)
Blend in a Vitamix blender with the plunger (use the plunger aggressively). Serve with cacao nibs sprinkled on top.
Serves 4
Smile and enjoy!

Cashew Cream Dessert (Jennifer Bodaken)

½ cup cashews
4 dates
2/3 cup cold water
8 ice cubes (optional)

Vitamix first three ingredients and then add four ice cubes and blend again. Serve chilled.

For vanilla cashew cream, add 1 tsp vanilla (or vanilla powder) and use orange juice instead of water.

Resources

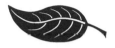

A Well Fed World: Feeding families / Saving animals. **awfw.org**

Sea Shepherd Conservation Society: Marine wildlife conservation organization. **seashepherd.org**

Nutritionfacts.org: Nutrition related research by Dr. Michael Greger M.D. **nutritionfacts.org**

Physicians Committee for Responsible Medicine: Physicians dedicated to improving people's health through a plant-based diet. **pcrm.org**

Farm Sanctuary: Farm animal shelters working to end stop animal cruelty. **farmsanctuary.org**

Vegan 1 Day: Inspiring others to go vegan one day at a time. **vegan1day.org**

Food For Life Global: World's largest vegan-veg food relief. **ffl.org**

Chooseveg.com: Comprehensive guide to vegan information. **chooseveg.com**

Vegan.com: Guide to going vegan. **vegan.com**

Our Hen House: Multi media outlet changing the world for animals. **ourhenhouse.org**

Herbivore Clothing Co.: Cruelty-free culture, fashion, books, etc. **herbivoreclothing.com**

Animal Place: Farm animal rescue - sanctuary. **animalplace.org**

We Animals: Documenting the lives of animals through photography. **weanimals.org**

Cowspiracy: Documentary movie about the environmental impacts of animal agriculture. **cowspiracy.com**

Forks Over Knives: Documentary movie about health benefits of a plant-based diet. **forksoverknives.com**

About the Authors

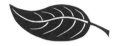

John Merryfield is a poet, surfer, SUP paddler, and painting contractor working out of Lake Tahoe, California. He is an ordinary guy with an extraordinary zeal for living life to the fullest. He is co-founder and director of the Vegan 1 Day Project, which is a grass-roots effort to encourage people to eat a plant-based diet. He divides his time between Lake Tahoe, California, and Los Barriles, Baja, Mexico. John has published poems to *Simply Haiku* journal and *Notes from the Gean* journal, as well as an awarded renku to the *Journal of Renga and Renku*. He has also published several articles about health, veganism, and animal rights to the *Elephant Journal*.

Carol Merryfield is a poet, owner of her business, The House Therapist, and a lover of all animals. She is passionate about living an authentic life and is committed to love and family. She is co-founder of the Vegan 1 Day Project. She is a New York Italian who now enjoys living in Lake Tahoe, California and Los Barriles, Baja, Mexico.

Acknowledgments

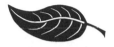

We would like to thank *A Well Fed World* and Dawn Moncrief for their support in writing this book.

The editing and insights we received from so many people were invaluable to us. Benjamin Allen's connection to the spirit of our lives and the message of our book was beyond measure. The contributions of Ed Bodaken, Heidi Pesterfield, Aaron Gottschalk, and Christina Shraefel were both generous and instrumental. Deborah Brown's creativity and her attention to the details were extraordinarily helpful.

We are continually inspired by people like Gene Baur, Rae Sikora, Will Tuttle, Jo-Anne McArthur, Nick Cooney, Bruce Friedrich, Paul Shapiro, Susie Coston, John Robbins, Mark Hawthorne and Erik Marcus and many others for their tireless efforts to create a more compassionate world.

To all who submitted recipes, we thank you for showing us what a compassionate kitchen looks like, and especially to Jennifer Bodaken, who has taught us so much about vegan cooking.

To the athletes who participate in our annual Vegan 1 Day event and potluck, Monica Quinones, Rob Gorder, Yolanda Labia, Billy Howard and so many more, thank you for always showing up.

We are indebted on a daily basis to the inspiration of our friends John Joseph, Jasmin Singer, Josh Hooten, Michelle Schwegmann, Keaven Van Lom, Alida Labia, Susan Kirkpatrick, Margaret Kirkpatrick, Aquila Nelson, Vee Lewin, and the entire Vegan 1 Day Community. Thanks for blazing a path and living a good life.

Advance Praise

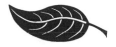

Vegan 1 Day is a beautiful testament to what we can do to make a difference and why it is so important to do so. Through the eyes and hearts of John and Carol we get to see how precious each day and each act is to the world within us and around us.

~ Benjamin Allen, author of *Out of the Ashes,*
Healing in the Afterloss

Part biography, part treatise on healthier living, *Vegan 1 Day* is a guide to a more compassionate, fulfilling existence. Infused with brief stories that reflect the authors' values and simple-but-satisfying plant-based recipes, this little book is sure to inspire readers to live ethically and with greater purpose.

~ Mark Hawthorne, author of three books on animal rights:
A Vegan Ethic: Embracing A Life Of Compassion Toward All,
Bleating Hearts: The Hidden World of Animal Suffering, and
Striking at the Roots: A Practical Guide to Animal Activism

Carol and John begin their lovely and lyrical book by reminding us, "We are capable of so much more than we allow." *Vegan 1 Day* can help each one of us live a fuller, more compassionate and beauty-filled life. I thank them for sharing their stories and allowing us to learn from their wisdom.

~ Jasmin Singer, co-founder of Our Hen House and
author of *Always Too Much and Never Enough*

Vegan 1 Day made my heart fill with joy. I couldn't wait to read each new chapter and hear what adventures John and Carol got into next. Yes, this short, thoughtful book is about living a life — even if just one day a week — that doesn't depend upon the intentional hurting and killing of thinking, feeling beings for every meal. It's described beautifully in the phrase "veganism is not a path of perfection, it's a path of kindness." But the book is also about a spiritual journey, one filled with moments like paddleboarding in the ocean and suddenly being surrounded by deadly orcas. Insights, missteps, compassion and good food are all described in a humble way that will make you want to share their stories and recipes.

~ Mark Robison, co-founder of Cockadoodlemoo
Farm Animal Sanctuary

36796324R00086

Made in the USA
San Bernardino, CA
02 August 2016